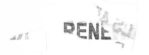

IN A WORLD OF
THEIR OWN

IN A WORLD OF THEIR OWN

EXPERIENCING UNCONSCIOUSNESS

Madelaine Lawrence

PRAEGER

Westport, Connecticut
London

Library of Congress Cataloging-in-Publication Data

Lawrence, Madelaine.
    In a world of their own : experiencing unconsciousness / Madelaine
Lawrence.
        p.   cm.
    Includes bibliographical references and index.
    ISBN 0–275–95323–8 (alk. paper)
    1. Coma. 2. Loss of consciousness. 3. Subconsciousness. 4. Near
-death experiences. I. Title.
    [DNLM: 1. Unconsciousness. 2. Death. WL 341 L422i 1997]
RB 150.C6L39   1997
616.8′49—dc20
DNLM/DLC
for Library of Congress   96–25076

British Library Cataloguing in Publication Data is available.

Library of Congress Catalog Card Number: 96–25076
ISBN: 0–275–95323–8

First published in 1997

Praeger Publishers, 88 Post Road West, Westport, CT 06881
An imprint of Greenwood Publishing Group, Inc.

Printed in the United States of America

∞™

The paper used in this book complies with the
Permanent Paper Standard issued by the National
Information Standards Organization (Z39.48–1984).

10 9 8 7 6 5 4 3 2 1

Copyright Acknowledgments

The author and publisher gratefully acknowledge permission to use the following
source:

Ring, K., and M. Lawrence (1993). Further evidence for veridical perception
during near-death experiences. *Journal of Near-Death Studies* (New York: Ple-
num Publishing), Summer, 223–229.

"I would not," says Socrates, "be confident in everything I say about the argument: but one thing I would fight for to the end, both in word or deed if I were able—that if we believed we should try to find out what is not known, we should be better and braver and less idle than if we believed that what we do not know is impossible to find out and that we need not even try."

—*The Meno*

CONTENTS

ACKNOWLEDGMENTS

The author wishes to thank the librarians at Robinson library at Hartford Hospital, the Eileen Garrett Library of the Parapsychology Foundation, Inc. in New York and the medical library at Middlesex Hospital for their extensive data searches.

Also greatly appreciated is the funding from the Research Office at Hartford Hospital, without whose help the project would not have been possible.

A thank you also is given to friends and family for their love and support during this entire book writing process.

IN A WORLD OF
THEIR OWN

1

INTRODUCTION

A young nursing student was assigned to care for a 45–year-old man who had brain surgery. The patient was unresponsive most of the time—just lying in bed or sitting in a chair, staring into space.

In spite of the lack of an overt response, the student had the sense that somehow there was communication. As the number of days she cared for him increased, she grew to notice some of his subtle expressions—even pain in his eyes. It seemed that when his wife came to visit, he moved more, his muscles strengthened, as if he were responding to her presence.

The patient and student developed a routine. When she explained what she was doing, he seemed to relax more. He would become agitated and restless when left in an uncomfortable position. She began to use these nonverbal cues to identify his needs. It would be an exaggeration to say that he anticipated her activities, but there seemed to be some awareness—some response to what she was doing for him.

His wife would visit daily and ask if he talked or responded differently in any way. The young student lacked the confidence to pass along her observations. The wife would talk about their life together, and all that they had once done. She looked for a sign that some of that previous life would return. The student nurse remained silent.

A few years later, our nursing student was a registered nurse working in an intensive care unit, caring for a young man on a ventilator. The patient, whose eyes were closed, was quite restless. He kept pulling at his restraints, tossing in bed. She and another nurse kept explaining what they were doing, trying to calm him down. As they suctioned him, he thrashed about, almost pulling off the restraints on his hands. He seemed frightened. He had tried to pull out his endotracheal tube (a tube placed in his trachea and attached to the ventilator to assist with breathing) several times before and they were afraid he'd try the same thing again. They were forced to sedate him further even though they knew that more narcotics would not help his physical condition. She kept thinking that there must be a better way.

Like most registered nurses, she had been taught to talk to unconscious patients, told that "hearing was the last sense to go." Although she did talk to her unconscious patients, she found it difficult to speak to someone who lay motionless and unresponsive. She kept looking for some sign that the person could hear.

In 1982, while I was working on my doctorate, my advisor suggested that I take one more graduate-level psychology class. After substantial resistance (I had already taken the required number of psychology courses at another university), I enrolled in a class on death and dying taught by Ken Ring. Ken was the author of *Life at Death: A Scientific Investigation of the Near-Death Experience*. Prior to this course, I was vaguely familiar with NDEs but had not paid much attention to them. During the class, however, I became fascinated with the stories that Ken and those whom he invited to class reported.

One subject, Carol, came to the class to talk about her near-death experience, giving us details of what she could hear and understand while the doctors and nurses attending her considered her to be "unconscious." She told of their comments that she would "probably not make it," and that, if she did, she would be "nothing more than a vegetable." I remember sitting in class thinking, "Oh, my God, she remembers what it was like to be unconscious."

As part of a course project I interviewed Carol for more details about her experience. While the members of the medical profession caring for her had thought that she was "out of it," in reality, she could hear their conversations. She also said she could feel her husband's anger and hostility—and that it caused her to retreat even further into her unconsciousness. Unknown to her family, friends, and the medical professionals, she was far from unaware. While they thought she was experiencing nothing, she was receiving a flood of data and emotions that would make a lifelong impact on her.

My reluctance at being in the class changed to enthusiasm, and I diligently researched the literature about unconsciousness. There were considerable written works on the physiology of the brain and the pathophysiology of the numerous conditions causing unconsciousness or coma. However, virtually nothing had been recorded describing the patient's experience in this state.

Carol's story, and the experiences of others I had observed as a young student and nurse, motivated me to continue my observation of unconscious patients with a research study of the experiences undergone by these patients. As I conducted my interviews, I learned that some people who became unconscious during incidents that did not draw them near to death—for instance, childbirth—also had intriguing stories to tell. One woman, for example, had an out-of-body experience (OBE) during a difficult labor.

This book is based on the research I conducted over a ten-year period. During the first phase, the pilot study, I interviewed 11 patients, talked to about a dozen doctors and nurses, and reviewed case studies in the literature and the library of the International Association of Near-Death Studies (IANDS). Patients from the pilot study were selected because they were willing to participate, having been referred to me by colleagues and friends.

During the second phase, at Hartford Hospital, a major teaching facility in Connecticut, I was able to interview over a hundred patients who had recently recovered from an unconscious experience. This was a descriptive study with both qualitative and quantitative components, focusing on the states that patients experience while unresponsive and the consistent themes, patterns, and characteristics of these states.

Most of the subjects I studied at Hartford Hospital were identified through weekly unit rounds. In some cases, I sent letters to patients who had been discharged, informing them of the research and inviting them to take part. All subjects had documented episodes of unconsciousness. Subjects with a documented history of a psychiatric illness were excluded from the study. A taped interview and medical chart audit were conducted for each subject. In the interview, I asked the subjects to describe the last thing they remembered before becoming unconscious. That question enabled me to determine the subjects' perception of when they were unaware or had been perceived to be unaware. I would then encourage them to elaborate on what they heard, saw, felt, and thought. From the charts, I obtained information about the subjects' diagnosis, how they came to be unconscious, the length of time they were observed to be unconscious, and any descriptions of them in this state.

Whenever possible, I interviewed a family member or a member of the staff who also observed the unconscious state. In most cases, I interviewed the patients within days of their unconscious experiences. There were some subjects whom I did not reach until almost a year had elapsed. In a very few instances, I talked with people many years after the event. At times, people described not only recent but past experiences as well.

In order to provide confidentiality the names and identifying characteristics of the subjects were changed. Any similarities to other persons are unintentional.

I tried to control for overrepresentation of unusual experiences through systematic rounds in the intensive care units (ICUs) and step-down units. However, many nurses and doctors at Hartford Hospital were aware of my research, and even though I told them that I was interested in interviewing any former *unconscious* patients, they had a tendency to refer to me those people who had *unusual* experiences.

PROCEDURES

Data were collected during face-to-face interviews, which were taped and transcribed. Van Kaam's phenomenological method was used to guide data collection and analysis. Subjects were encouraged to lead the interview and give an undirected account of their experiences.

Phenomenology is both a philosophy and a research methodology. In both regards, the phenomenologist gives primacy to the experience of the individual, which was the way I conducted this study. Phenomenology is the study of the lived experience. This research was the study of the lived experience of being unconscious. The perceptions of the individual, accurate or false, are what matter, since it is the person's perception that governs his or her behavior, beliefs, and values.

Phenomenologists are divided concerning the ultimate use of the data. Some believe phenomenological reports should contain only the stories of the lived experiences of the subjects. These research reports read like nonfiction novels. The reader feels an affinity for the subjects and understands and appreciates through insights the subject's point of view and experiences during a certain life experience.

Other phenomenologists, of which I consider myself one, value the insight and understanding of the human experience but also support the analysis of the components of the experiences and the confirmation of the experience through other data sources. The analysis includes a breakdown of the components of the experience into concepts and hypotheses. The concepts are compared to results from other studies. Confirmation is obtained through a process referred to as triangulation, in which additional data are collected through other means, methods, or researchers. In this study, the chart audits and interviews with significant others or staff who were present during the unconscious episodes constituted the triangulation methods. All the data were compared with consistency, and inconsistencies were noted. In this research, there was considerable inconsistency, for example, between the subjects' descriptions of when they were unconscious and the perceptions of the caregivers.

To date, the study includes 111 patients: 11 from the pilot and the remaining from the Hartford Hospital study. What is published here are the results of the study, known similar reported experiences, and possible explanations of the phenomena described. Of the one hundred people I interviewed from Hartford Hospital, one in four (27%) had no recollection of any experience during unconsciousness. Nine percent fell into the category of inner awareness—experiencing emotions while unconscious and yet receiving no stimuli from the external environment.

Twenty-seven percent of the patients went through the phase of perceived unconsciousness. During this state those around them believed that they were completely unaware while they were, in fact, hearing sounds and/or experiencing tactile sensations when they were moved or prodded. Fourteen percent of those in the study underwent distorted consciousness and experienced hallucinations, memory lapses, and personality changes. As mentioned previously, one in four (23%) of those interviewed told me about some sort of extrasensory event that they had encountered during their unconsciousness (Table 1.1). In a few cases subjects experienced more than one type of state.

Table 1.1
Five States of Altered Consciousness Experiences

1. Unconsciousness (27%)

2. Perceived Unconsciousness (27%)
   Auditory
   Tactile
   Emotional
   Motion

3. Inner Awareness (9%)

4. Distorted consciousness (14%)
   Perception distortion
   Memory distortion
   Personality distortion

5. Extrasensory Experiences (23%)
   Out-of-body experiences
   Near-death experiences
   Near-death visits
   Encounters with the grim reaper

Of the total subjects studied from both the pilot study and the Hartford Hospital study, the mean age was 57, with actual ages ranging from 21 to 83. Sixty-four percent of the subjects were male and 36 percent were female. The majority of the patients (68%) had some form of heart disease. Patients with heart disease tend to have frequent unconscious episodes from which they recover completely. Eleven percent of the patients had head injuries, 6 percent some neurovascular disorder, 4.5 percent had diabetes, 4.5 percent had seizures, and 6 percent had miscellaneous causes of their unconsciousness. Table 1.2 contains the breakdown of the five states according to age, gender, and diagnosis.

This book is organized in accordance with the type of experiences patients have and the descriptions of major paradigms, theories, and assumptions commonly used to explain those experiences. Chapters 2, 3, and 9 contain historical perspectives on the major research paradigms in the fields that have attempted to explain the phenomena experienced by these unconscious patients. Each subsequent chapter also includes research related to that particular state.

This book is also organized in a way that addresses both phenomenological points of view. Chapter 4 is Carol's story, part of which I first heard in the class taught by Ken Ring. Because she experienced so many of the states of consciousness described by the patients, her story gives a wonderful example of what a lived experience of unconsciousness is for a patient. Most of the remaining chapters describe experiences of individuals who primarily experienced only one state. In fact, most patients only experienced one or two states while unconscious.

There are four major points in the book. First, it is recognized that unconsciousness is a state of living and not just emptiness. Second, these experiences have a profound effect on the person. Third, some of the experiences are not explainable by science as we know it. Fourth, our progress in understanding these experiences seems to be impeded by our compartmentalization of the study of man through different disciplines and by the restraints imposed by religion and society to study experiences that are labeled as extrasensory or soul-like phenomena.

Table 1.2
Hartford Hospital Study

State	M	Age	F	M	Diagnosis
Unconsciousness	27	60	9	18	Cardiac = 21 Head injuries = 3 Diabetes = 2 Miscellaneous = 1
Perceived Unconsciousness	27	60	13	14	Cardiac = 19 Cerebral hemorrhage = 1 Head Injury = 2 Seizures = 2 Miscellaneous = 3
Inner Awareness	9	56	3	6	Cardiac = 9
Distorted Consciousness	14	52	3	11	Cardiac = 5 Head injuries = 4 Seizures = 2 Cerebral hemorrhage = 2 Diabetes = 1 Miscellaneous = 2
Extrasensory	23	58	9	14	Cardiac = 7 Head injury = Cerebral hemorrhage = 2 Diabetes = 1 Miscellaneous = 2

OVERVIEW

Although this book is directed by the results of the research that I have personally conducted, it often contains references to other studies and theories that have arisen from the research done on unconsciousness and near-death experiences. The primary goal of this work, however, is to relate the stories of those who have undergone events totally unlike anything they had previously experienced in their lives. It is also the goal of this book to help the reader to experience what a patient may live through while unconscious: the confusion, pleasure, fear, and excitement a person can have in the various states we refer to as unconsciousness. I hope these patient experiences can be used to promote better understanding of the needs of patients in these states.

2

HISTORICAL THEORIES, ASSUMPTIONS, AND BELIEFS

After conducting and analyzing the interviews that are described in this book, I looked for greater understanding and explanations of these experiences described by the subjects but found that no one theory nor any one discipline's paradigm satisfactorily explains them. In fact, there is a considerable battle raging among the disciplines to explain similar experiences, each believing its point of view is the correct one.

This chapter, along with Chapters 3 and 9, is intended to provide a brief overview of some of the paradigms and assumptions put forth in history by various disciplines to explain the relationships between the body, mind, and soul (Hunt, 1993). These chapters provide background information for understanding how various disciplines view these experiences and should also prepare the reader for the related research studies at the end of each chapter of patient experiences.

The patient experiences described in this book are addressed primarily by medical science (which includes medicine and nursing), psychology, parapsychology, and physics. This chapter describes scientific paradigms and presents information on the historical assumptions and beliefs about the mind, body, and soul and how they still influence our present disciplines. Chapter 3 prepares one for the first four patient experiences: unconsciousness, inner awareness, perceived unconsciousness, and distorted consciousness. Those experiences are addressed primarily by medical science, psychology, and physics, whose major points of view are described.

Chapter 9 describes primarily the assumptions of parapsychology since the patient phenomona (out-of-body, near-death experiences, near-death visits, and apparitions of the grim reaper) discussed in Chapters 10 through 13 are primarily studied by that discipline.

SCIENTIFIC PARADIGMS

Some of the greatest insights into the development of science are contained in a small book, *The Structure of Scientific Revolutions,* written by Thomas Kuhn in 1970. Kuhn, an observer of the development of many disciplines, sees us—and scientists, in particular—as being governed by paradigms. Kuhn defined a paradigm as the patterns of assumptions, methods, and theories that organize the development of knowledge in a discipline. These patterns influence how we view the world. Once we know and accept the paradigm, the world becomes organized for us. We understand how the components fit together and the rules that govern the processes inherent in our world. Paradigms are very important in maintaining order and stability and the promotion of the development of what Kuhn calls normal science.

Normal science proceeds by creating theories and hypotheses as well as conducting studies that fit within the assumptions of the current paradigm. These studies and this incremental growth fill in the unknown portions of the paradigm. We assume, for example, that humans have needs and carry out a number of roles. Scientists who study in these areas then proceed to identify types of human needs and roles, what circumstances influence individuals in having certain needs and selecting certain roles. The opportunities for research on human needs and roles are almost endless. The theories, assumptions, and methods of the study of these phenomena soon become a well established part of the paradigm and the normal science of that discipline.

Theories become an important part of the discipline. They are necessary to help us understand and organize facts. In 1904, the physicist W. F. Barrett wrote: "Without a theory facts are a mob, not an army." A theory in its simplest form is a number of concepts whose relationships are described by propositions. Abraham Maslow's hierarchy of needs is a good example. Maslow defined a number of concepts known as needs: physiological, safety, social, self-esteem, and self-actualization. Just identifying these needs is not enough to call these statements a theory. Maslow also proposed certain relationships relative to these needs: there is an order to the needs, the basic needs have to be met before a person can move up to the next level of needs, and fewer individuals will meet the higher level needs, than the basic ones.

Theories are neither facts nor proven statements. They are ideas or insights about relationships that need to be tested. Some theories like Maslow's hierarchy of needs are easily grasped and intuitively understood by most people. Others like Einstein's theory of relativity are highly complex and understood primarily by experts in the field—and sometimes even then in limited numbers. Theories make scientific information more easily understood and meaningful. They give us a framework for understanding phenomena and situations. Maslow's theory, for example, would enable us to decide how to help someone who had low self esteem. If that person was hungry and in an unsafe environment, we would be better advised to help him meet those needs first before working on self-esteem needs.

To be accepted, theories should be tested and validated through research. This testing is part of the normal science process. Some disciplines are more or less theoretical, and some disciplines test and develop theories more than others.

Each discipline follows rules and assumptions they have developed to guide scientific inquiry. In general, scientists develop:

1. Acceptable theories or concepts
2. Acceptable methodology
3. Prescribed rules of evidence
4. Hypotheses or research questions about the context of the phenomenon

William Harman also describes the metaphysical foundations of modern science as being either objective, positivist, or reductionist. He defines these words in the following way:

> Objectivism: the assumption of an objective world which the observer can hold at a distance and study separately from himself.
> Positivism: the assumption that the real world is what is physically measurable.
> Reductionism: the assumption that we come to really understand a phenomenon through studying the behavior of its elemental parts (e.g., fundamental particles). (Harman, 1991, p. 14)

Paradigms and assumptions and guides like those described can hinder as well as help the development of an area of knowledge. Kenneth Pelletier points out the deficiencies of a paradigm in the following way; "The paradigm dictates the essence of the questions to be raised and the means by which they are resolved. The paradigm itself is never questioned. In this sense, paradigms serve as prisms directing the attention of researchers only to the groupings and correlations of data that lend themselves to that particular kind of investigation" (Pelletier, 1985, pp. 37–38).

In fact, scientists can become blinded by the restraints put on them by their paradigms. Kuhn, however, describes how knowledge develops in spite of the paradigm in vogue at the time. Science also develops, according to Kuhn, by undergoing revolutions in these underlying paradigms. This development begins with anomalies that are no longer explained by the old paradigm and theories. The women's movement, for example, challenged many of the well-established beliefs about the roles women could engage in. The old paradigm included assumptions about women that today are unthinkable. For example, women were not allowed to be school bus drivers, police detectives, or pilots. There were very few women doctors and lawyers. The few women who somehow took on these roles initially were exceptions but eventually showed that the assumptions of the old paradigm could not satisfactorily explain their satisfaction and success in roles that the old paradigm said could only be carried out by men.

As with most revolutions, scientific revolutions are not easy. There is an initial attempt by some members of the established science to consciously or unconsciously deny the existence of the anomalies because the influence of the paradigm is so strong. Even before the women's movement, young girls and young women did as well as their male counterparts in school, but those occurrences did not eliminate the belief that women should not be prepared for intellectually challenging careers. They were filtered. Because paradigms are so integrated into what we consider to be normal, they are very difficult to even recognize, never mind change. This change often comes about when someone comes from a different paradigm and has the courage to face the resistance that almost always occurs.

There is initially an attempt to hold on to the old theories of the old paradigm to explain the anomalies. Often scientists have devoted much of their professional life to testing certain theories and refining them. To be presented now with an anomaly that, in effect, says that their theories are incorrect is a difficult situation to accept. Sometimes this resistance is minor; sometimes it is life threatening. It is not unusual for someone who is advocating something that will result in a new paradigm to be laughed at or even discredited. Eventually, as the paradigm shifts and new information becomes available through research, theories are altered and sometimes discarded (Table 2.1).

Table 2.1
An Outline of the Development of the Study of the Mind, Body, Self, and Soul of Man

A. The nature of man examined philosophically

B. Man divided into body, mind, and soul through philosophical inquiry

C. Disciplines that study different dimensions of man develop separate from each other
   1. Medical science
      a. body and brain explained by physical sciences
      b. some recognition of the influence of emotions on health of the body
      c. psychiatry describes the effects of emotional trauma
   2. Psychology
      a. mind and self become phenomena for scientific inquiry
      b. behavior and mental processes the focus
   3. Parapsychology
      a. began survival research
      b. acceptance of the possibility of extrasensory experiences
   4. Quantum physics
      a. integration of particles and waves
      b. describe a space-time continuum

HISTORICAL PARADIGMS

Centuries ago there was not a great distinction made between the body, the mind, the self, and the spirit or soul of man. Early in our civilization we attributed many events or experiences to higher beings. Illness or wellbeing, for example, was the result of God's (or gods') being pleased or displeased with our behavior.

Hippocrates (460–377), the father of medicine, was the first to significantly divorce medicine from religion and superstition. He proposed that all diseases had natural causes and were not the work of the gods. He taught that most of the physical and mental illnesses had a physical basis. However, he incorrectly assumed this physical basis to be part of a four-element theory: earth, air, fire, and water. He believed good health was the balance of these elements, and for centuries physicians would try to treat these imbalances by draining procedures, like bloodletting, or additive procedures like administering herbs and drugs whose purpose was to add substances that were lacking (Hunt, 1993).

Socrates (469–399) was a contemporary of Hippocrates and a well-respected philosopher. He contributed to the initial description of the properties of the mind by pointing out our ability to reason. By questioning, he led his pupils to the answers they sought. His deductive, inference-by-inference questioning led us to believe that knowledge exists within us. Another major contribution from Socrates was his inference that the existence of innate knowledge proved that we possessed an immortal soul, which was an entity that could exist apart from the brain and body. Hippocrates and Socrates laid the foundation for considering how the body, mind, and soul were at times separate and at times together (Hunt, 1993).

Plato (447–327), the most famous pupil of Socrates, was a dualist who believed in the separation of the body from the mind and soul. He saw the soul as not only an immortal entity but also as mind. It was his belief that the soul was behind thought or reason, spirit or will, and appetite or desire, although he never explained how thinking can take place in a nonmaterial essence. He also believed that the highest goal of the soul was to escape from the body, which he considered bonds of matter.

Aristotle (384–322), Plato's most distinguished pupil, divided knowledge into two distinct categories. There were physical and nonphysical aspects of reality, physics and metaphysics. Aristotle believed that the soul was the essence of the body and represented our individuality. He used the term psyche to mean the entire soul or occasionally just the part of the soul where thinking takes place. Aristotle was monistic in his views, believing that the soul or psyche was not an entity that could exist apart from the body (Hunt, 1993).

After Hippocrates, Socrates, Plato, and Aristotle there was a long dormant period before philosophers and scientists again addressed the nature of man. It was commonly believed that these famous thinkers had given the world the answers to the understanding of man and that no further exploration was necessary. Their positions and beliefs were not greatly expanded upon until St. Augustine (354–430) and St. Thomas Aquinas (1225–1274). Augustine and Thomas Aquinas became speakers representing the strong influence that Catholicism had on science and the study of the body, mind, and soul.

Augustine described the three functions of the mind: memory, reason, and will. He primarily supported Plato's belief that the soul is immortal and survives the death of the body. He believed, however, that during the time it was part of the body, the soul was also the mind. He supported the primacy of the belief in scripture and religious doctrine. Science was good only when it served religious purposes.

Thomas Aquinas supported the notion of a soul-body unit during life and the belief that the soul lives on after death. He also further defined the functions of the psyche, Aristotle's soul-mind, into the vegetative or autonomic functions, sentient (perception, appetite, and locomotion) and the rational or reason and memory functions. He is truly the forerunner of our approach to studying the subfunctions of the brain (Hunt, 1993).

Rene Descartes (1596–1650) is considered to be one of the most influential philosophers of the modern era. As part of his search to describe the nature of man, Descartes supported the division of man into two parts: the body and the mind. His famous saying "Cognito ergo sum" (I think therefore I am) reinforced the belief that mind and body were separate. Wanting to stay on good terms with the Catholic church, Descartes also taught that what was acceptable for scientific study were only those objects clearly visible and in public space. Things of thought were located in private space not suitable for scientific study but rather the purview of religious authority. Science then was limited to the study of the nature of man through the study of the body or objective reality only.

The fifteenth century thus became a turning point for the development of science. Descartes's support of Rome simultaneously freed and enslaved us. The influence of religious authorities on the study of objective reality was now loosened. Previously the Greek astronomers had established the belief that the earth was the center of the universe. The religious authorities viewed this belief as consistent with their view that God was the ultimate mover of the earth. Earth's central position reaffirmed the belief in man as being the masterpiece of God's creation (Damasio,1994).

Galileo, in later years, broke new ground with his ability to "see the heavens" more clearly with his telescope. Since he could see more than Aristotle was able to, he knew that Aristotle could not have known all there was to know. Galileo published and talked about his theories and fundamentally supported Copernicus, proving Aristotle wrong. His findings were also inconsistent with religious beliefs. In 1633 Galileo was tried before the Inquisition and told to publically renounce his support of the Copernican theory.

The church by that time was not the influential force it once had been. In 1520 it had faced a major rift when the German cleric Martin Luther was excommunicated by Pope Leo X. The Christian world had become divided into Protestant and Roman Catholic. It was in this revolutionary atmosphere that the revolution in man's ideas began. The Protestant countries became less worried about the theory of a central earth. There was a growing body of scientifically minded individuals who saw the role of science as separate from the role of religion. There was also now a challenge to the beliefs and assumptions of Socrates, Plato, and Aristotle. It became clear there was more to know about human nature than these great philosophers had been able to describe.

It was also during this time that the study of accurate anatomy and physiology began. Four hundred years before, Galen had described the body as containing a rudimentary circulatory system very much influenced by spirits: the vital spirit, the natural spirit, and the animal spirit. By contrast, William Harvey (1578–1657) described how the heart circulates the blood around the body, a function no longer attributed to spirits (Hunt, 1993). These scientific discoveries successfully challenged the beliefs of orthodox religion on objective reality. According to Pelletier, "Science offered man visible, testable and observable proof rather than faith, dogma and oppressive liturgical hierarchy. Over the centuries science came to displace religious dogma as the basis of a comprehensive and compelling belief system" (Pelletier, 1985, p. 13).

While man was now free to study the physical world and body, the soul or mind was not subjected to scientific inquiry. Religious authorities still claimed those dimensions of man as their exclusive province. Mind was avoided by classical science as a topic for research because it was not seen as physical and also not seen as capable of being studied experimentally. Because science was still young and developing, scientists felt the need to disassociate themselves from anything remotely religious or mystical in order to be recognized as scientific, since religion was equated with faith and science with reason.

Also, the separation of physical and nonphysical reality initiated a compartmental approach to the study of the mind, body, and soul and the development of various disciplines to study components of nature and man. This led for the first time to a nonholistic approach to the study of the nature of man.

Pelletier describes this compartmentalization well by discussing how different disciplines might view the problem "How do I move my arm?" He believes, "A biochemist will explore the actin-myosin process in muscular contraction; a biophysicist may use a scanning election microscope to observe the molecular and atomic structures involved in movement; while a psychologist may seek the motivation for such an act in terms of a response to a set of particular internal or external stimuli. Whatever the case may be, each scientist is trained to state and study the problem in terms of the rules of evidence and methods of inquiry appropriate to his training" (Pelletier, 1985, p. 40).

The next chapter describes the development of the underlying assumptions of the various disciplines and how some of these historical beliefs still provide the underpinnings for their paradigms.

NOTE

Much of the research for this chapter relied on Hunt, M. (1993). *The Story of Psychology*. New York: Anchor Books.

3

PARADIGMS OF THE DISCIPLINES: MEDICAL SCIENCE, PSYCHOLOGY, PARAPSYCHOLOGY, AND PHYSICS

MEDICAL SCIENCE

The methods used by medical science to study the body have been seen as primarily objective and reductionistic. Medical science is greatly influenced by two of the beliefs of our current scientific method: the notion that greater understanding is obtained by reducing what we see to the basic elements of the phenomena, and that knowing through sense experience, unassisted or assisted with instruments, constitutes proof.

In medical science the body is seen as having different parts and different functions, most of which could be described by the anatomy, physiology, and pathophysiology of a particular segment of the body. Lacking the integration of the study of the nonobservable components of human nature like emotions and appreciation, the methods of inquiry seem cold and clinical. There are some authors who go so far as to refer to the methods used in medical science as the "body shop" approach, studying and treating a person in a way a mechanic would repair a car.

The brain also has become a specialized area of study. The brain, as we now understand it, is believed to have evolved over a period of millions of years. Four general types of functions have been described, two having to do with survival and two with more creative processes. The survival functions include arousal and wakefulness associated with the brain stem, and emotions and the inner state of the body associated with the limbic system. The creative processes include learning, memory, and perception associated with the cortex, and language and art associated with the divided hemispheres.

In medical science the study of consciousness is focused primarily on wakefulness and rudimentary cognitive mental functions. A person is considered conscious if he or she is alert and oriented to time, person, and place, thus alert enough to hear and respond to questions and possessing cognitive functioning sufficient to answer the questions.

Early researchers established the importance of the role of the brainstem in providing the mechanism for wakefulness in humans (Berger in 1929 and Bremer in 1936). Other researchers identified ascending, nonspecific mechanisms in the brainstem that influenced arousal, later referred to as the reticular activating system (RAS) (Morrison and Dempsey in 1942).

The reticular formation is the central core of the brainstem comprised of two structures, the medulla and the thalamus. This system is stimulated by every major somatic and special sensory pathway. The RAS controls our ability to be awake, to sleep, and to pay attention. The cerebral cortex is stimulated by and in turn innervates the reticular formation. There is a major feedback mechanism between the RAS and cerebral cortex by which incoming information is regulated. The integration of the reticular formation with the cerebral cortex enables us not only to be aware but also to understand what is happening in our environment.

The limbic system, which comprises a border of cellular structures between the brain stem and the cortex, helps us maintain homeostasis. Emotions are controlled within this limbic system. It is believed that emotional needs as well as basic physiological and safety needs are given primacy over consciousness. It is difficult to think clearly, for example, when under the influence of strong emotions.

The brain in all primates is divided into hemispheres. Only human brains, however, have hemispheres specialized for different functions. Roger Sperry, a neurophysiologist, did extensive experimentation on brain functioning of laboratory animals and described the unique functions of each cerebral hemisphere in humans. The left hemisphere was found to govern the right side of the body and to be the analytical, rational, intellectual side of the human brain concerned with verbal and mathematical abstractions. The right hemisphere, which governs the left side of the body, controls more of the intuitive, holistic, and spatial tasks and enables us to appreciate music, recognize faces, and be spatially oriented. (For more detailed information about Sperry's findings, the reader is encouraged to pursue his publications cited in the reference list.)

It is common in medical practice to anticipate patient deficits based on the location of a brain growth or injury or defect. Medical science has shown through animal experiments and human occurrences that certain injuries, certain surgical interventions, or stimulation to various parts of the brain lead to certain reactions and/or deficits. Direct damage to the brain can alter a person's consciousness, through either direct external trauma or increased intracranial pressure. The brain can be severely affected by the swelling that results from constriction of the skeletal structure surrounding it, and because of the swelling, a person's consciousness is altered.

Sections I and II from Table 3.1 illustrate the common causes of unconsciousness or coma, including those caused by anatomical damage. Most medical textbooks will describe the type of consciousness deficits expected to be seen with the various types of lesions. Most physicians believe that damage to the brain is permanent. If there is any improvement to the person's ability to function, it is due to other parts of the brain taking over those lost functions.

Table 3.1
Cause of Stupor or Coma in Five Hundred Patients Initially Diagnosed as "Coma of Unknown Etilogy"

I. Supratentorial Lesions
   A. Rhinencephalic and subcortical destructive lesions
      1. thalamic infarcts
   B. Supratentorial mass lesions
      1. hemorrhage
         a. intracerebral
            (1) hypertensive
            (2) vascular anomaly
            (3) other
         b. epidural
         c. subdural
         d. pituitary apoplexy
      2. infarction
         a. arterial occlusions
            (1) thrombotic
            (2) embolic
         b. venous occlusions
      3. tumors
         a. primary
         b. metastatic
      4. abscess
         a. intracerebral
         b. subdural
      5. closed head injury

II. Subtentorial Lesions
   A. Compressive lesions
      1. cerebellar hemorrhage
      2. posterior fossa subdural or extradual hemorrhage
      3. cerebellar infarct
      4. cerebellar tumor
      5. cerebellar abscess
      6. basilar aneurysm
   B. Destructive or ischemic lesions
      1. pontine hemorrhage
      2. brainstem infarct

Table 3.1 continued

      3. basilar migraine

      4. brainstem demyelination

III. Diffuse and/or Metabolic Dysfunction

    A. Diffuse intrinsic disorders of brain

      1. "encephalitis" or encephalomyelitis

      2. subarachnoid hemorrhage

      3. concussion and postictal states

      4. primary neuronal disorders

    B. Extrinsic and metabolic disorders

      1. anoxia or ischemia

      2. hypoglycemia

      3. nutritional

      4. hepatic encephalopathy

      5. uremia and dialysis

      6. pulmonary disease

      7. endocrine disorders (including diabetes)

      8. remote effects of cancer

      9. drug poisons

      10. ionic and acid-base disorders

      11. temperature regulation

      12. mixed or nonspecific metabolic coma

IV Psychiatric "Coma"

    A. Conversion reactions

    B. Depression

    C. Catatonic stupor

Modified from Plum and Posner, 1982, p. 2.

Neuropharmacologic Mechanisms in Consciousness

We also know through medical science that certain chemicals can influence our degree of wakefulness. Taking stimulants like caffeine and amphetamines helps us stay awake. Other drugs like cocaine, psychedelics, atropine, scopolamine, some antidepressants, barbiturates, alcohol, opiates, and other sedatives can lead to delirium, stupor, or coma (Plum and Posner, 1982, p. 242). Internally cholinergic drugs and those in the central monamine system like serotonin and noradrenaline produce behavioral arousal.

Oxygen and glucose imbalance also can play a part in consciousness. According to Plum and Posner, because the brain is nourished by oxygen, glucose, and many other body chemicals, its health and activity are directly related to the proper proportion of these substances. If the brain is deprived of oxygen—such as occasioned by a stroke—or diminishment of glucose—as in diabetes—it does not function properly. The results are often unconsciousness.

Oxygen is critical to brain function. According to Arthur Guyton, "Lack of blood flow to the brain for more than 5 to 10 minutes usually results in permanent mental impairment or even total destruction of the brain. Even though the heart should be revived, the person might die from the effects of brain damage or live with permanent mental impairment" (Guyton, 1991, p. 145). The one notable exception to this principle is cold temperatures. Hypothermia decreases a body's need for oxygen. Near-drowning victims in extremely cold waters have been known to survive and not suffer permanent brain damage even when they were without oxygen for more than 10 minutes.

For medical science, being able to explain the anatomy, physiology, and pathophysiology of consciousness and unconsciousness is sufficient to explain how we have thoughts. What we know from medical science is that interference with the normal functioning of the brain not only leads to altered consciousness but also changed personalities, such as those altered by frontal lobe lesions.

Not all medical science researchers or practitioners subscribe to the reductionistic and materialistic approach regarding the connection between mind and body. A growing number of researchers have documented the impact that emotions have on the body and consciousness. We know now that many physical illnesses—heart disease, asthma, hypertension, ulcers, to name a few—are greatly affected by the emotional state of the individual. We also know that some illnesses long attributed to emotional causes, like premenstrual syndrome, addictions, some psychiatric illnesses, have a physiological component. Section IV of Plum and Posner's table of coma causes lists the psychiatric illnesses that can cause loss of consciousness or coma.

Psychiatry

Psychiatry as a clinical specialty within medicine has as its primary focus the emotional component of human nature. Psychiatry began, according to Franz Alexander and Sheldon Selesnick, the first time someone listened to another person describe his or her emotional distress and provided support and assistance to that person. There have been three basic trends in psychiatric thought throughout the history of psychiatry: the magical approach, the organic approach, and the psychological approach. Those who subscribed to magical beliefs as causing mental illness described the role of God or gods and devils in bringing about the malaise. It was not uncommon early in our history for people to believe in a mysterious outside force that took over the body. Those who ascribed to the organic approach believed that life can be described and understood in terms of physics and chemistry. The psychological approach was promoted by psychiatrists who recognized the effects of emotional trauma on the psyche. William Cullen (1712–1790) was one of the first to develop a comprehensive classification of mental illnesses and to use the term neurosis. While he recognized that mental illnesses were not accompanied by fevers or localized pathology, he supported the belief that some type of physiological breakdown was involved. Benjamin Rush (1745–1813), often referred to as the founder of American psychiatry, believed that mental illness was due to congested blood in the brain. This condition could be relieved by rotary movement like that caused by the gyrating chair. Johann Christian Reil was a physician who represented the transition between the organic and psychological beliefs in the causes of mental illnesses. He published the first systematic treatise on psychotherapy in 1803. He believed there was a close relationship between body and mind. "Feelings and ideas, psychic influences, are the proper means by which disturbances of the brain can be corrected and its vitality can be un-blocked" (Alexander and Selesnick, 1966, p. 136).

One of the most famous physicians who believed in the psycho-logical theories of mental illness was, of course, Sigmund Freud. Freud was born in 1856 in a small town in the Austro-Hungarian Empire. He graduated from medical school in 1881 after a six-year hiatus from school to study in a physiological institute. After postgraduate education, he entered into private practice as a neu-rologist in Vienna. In that practice he was referred patients who had neurological symptoms that could not be treated by conventional methods. It was through his work with these patients who saw snakes, rats, and vultures and who developed paralysis and antiso-cial behaviors that he eventually came to describe his theories and treatments of the unconscious mind.

Freud believed the mind had three levels of functioning: the conscious, the preconscious, and the unconscious. The unconscious he saw as containing powerful primitive drives and forbidden desires. These drives and desires motivated and influenced human behavior, often in an altered or disguised form. He also described how previous psychologically traumatic experiences influenced current behavior. His contributions to psychiatry and psychology have been delineated in the following way:

1883–1897, anatomy of the nervous system

1886–1895, studies in hypnotism and hysteria

1895–1920, demonstration and study of unconscious phenomena and the development of the psychoanalytic method of treatment

1920–1937, systematic inquiries into human personality (Alexander and Selesnick, 1966, p. 188)

Freud had a contemporary, Carl Jung, who devoted himself to psychoanalytic practice and activities. Jung would frequently con-verse with Freud and argue and occasionally disagree with Freud's interpretation of cases. Even though Jung was a physician he found more followers among nonpsychiatrists. He established training centers that accepted nonmedical candidates. His strong influence in psychology is described later in this chapter.

The development of medicine as a discipline was influenced strongly by the biomedical model. While the development of psychiatry included more concern about the mind and emotions of the individual, it also was and still is ambivalent about the role of physical causes and psychological trauma in precipitating mental illness. Such is not the case with the nursing profession.

Nursing

Nursing as a formal discipline began in the late nineteenth century. Florence Nightingale is credited as being the founder of the profession, although she was far from typical of the women who would become nurses. The early nurses were often women from religious orders or women from low socioeconomic classes. Nursing at its very beginning included a holistic and caring framework. As the professionals who spent the most time with the ill patient, nurses became more focused on the psychological as well as physical needs of the ill patients. Although initially trained in hospitals and currently educated in colleges and universities as well, they were and still are required to take liberal arts as well as science courses. Initially seen as an extension of male physicians, early in their history nurses sought autonomy in the psychosocial dimensions of patient care, dimensions not of particular interest to their medical colleagues. With many of the early nurses coming from religious orders and subsequent nurses identifying themselves as having strong religious beliefs, the spiritual and psychosocial domain was a natural area of focus.

Nursing, however, has been strongly influenced by the physiological tenets of medicine and has borrowed from that discipline and others like psychology to identify core theories and research methodologies. It was not until nursing education became college based in the 1960s that nursing began to develop its own theoretical base. Many of the early nurse theorists looked at human needs as a framework for organizing the developing knowledge in the discipline. Others looked at care deficits and how patients adapted.

Unique in the nursing profession was Martha Rogers' "Science of Unitary Human Beings." She described her works as basic science and not an application model. Her belief was that man is an energy field and as such interacts with the environment, which is also comprised of energy fields. Her theories influenced the development of therapeutic touch, described by Delores Krieger. Therapeutic touch was seen as a method of assessing and rebalancing the energy fields of a person. Never actually touching the person, the nurse moves her hands over the patient, feeling the energy and, through intense concentration, sending positive energy. Considerable research has been done on this technique. In one impressive study it was shown that therapeutic touch actually increased the hemoglobin levels of the patients receiving it. Not well accepted in the established health care community, nurses practice therapeutic touch and other alternative methods behind closed curtains (Rogers, 1986).

Nurses recognized that many symptoms associated with illness are influenced by psychological as well as physiological factors. Since they are with the patient, administering the medications, they can see that anxiety increases pain. It is no longer acceptable for nurses to simply medicate a patient for pain. It is just as important to help the patient identify underlying anxiety associated with the illness. The profession takes much more of an integrated mind-body approach to caring for the ill.

PSYCHOLOGY: THE STUDY OF THE MIND AND THE SELF

Some members of this discipline are not convinced that the physiological framework presented by medical science is adequate for explaining consciousness. Some humanistic psychologists, particularly, believe that medical science can explain the hardware of consciousness by describing the functions of the brain but not the software of consciousness, mind, and emotions. So, even though the exterior or body of the person is affected, that doesn't necessarily explain the inner workings of an individual. Software cannot be used when the hardware is broken, but that does not mean the software does not exist or could not be used under different circumstances.

Daniel Dennett, author of many books on consciousness and the director of the Center for Cognitive Studies at Tufts University, describes what is missing in the medical model:

> It seems that no mere machine, no matter how accurately it mimicked the brain processes . . . , would be capable of appreciating a wine, or a Beethoven sonata, or a basketball game. For appreciation you need consciousness—something no mere machine has. But of course the brain is a machine of sorts, an organ like the heart or lungs or kidneys with an ultimately mechanical explanation of all its powers. This can make it seem compelling that the brain isn't what does the appreciating: that is the responsibility (or privilege) of the mind. Reproduction of the brain's machinery in a silicon-based machine wouldn't, then, yield real appreciation, but at best the illusion or simulance of appreciation. (Dennett, 1991, p. 31)

Occurring parallel to the development of medical science was the development of psychology, often described as the science of mental life, including the study of feelings, desires, cognition, reasoning, decision making, and so forth. The study of the mind began in the nineteenth century as the discipline of psychology. Most authorities agree that psychology started in 1879, in the laboratory of a middle-aged professor named Wilhelm Wundt and two of his students. This was the first psychology experiment conducted in a laboratory. An experimental approach to the study of the mind was thought to be the most scientific. Mindful of the history of the influence of the church and in their desire to be scientific, questions of spirit and divinity were left closeted. Materialistic tendencies prevailed. Although psychologists were supposedly studying the psyche, Aristotle's notion that the mind was also influenced by the spirit was eliminated. Many psychologists believed that all mental functions were essentially neural processes and that the mind only existed as part of the body.

Psychology, however, became a diverse discipline and no one fundamental belief or assumption prevailed. Some psychologists followed the path of physiology or behaviorism, objectifying all components of mind and consciousness. The German physiological psychologists of the late nineteenth and early twentieth centuries, for example, believed that all mental conditions were nothing but physiological states of the brain and nervous system. Their contemporary supporter, Francis Crick, describes consciousness as "a continuous, semi-oscillatory firing of sets of neurons" (Crick, 1994). Likewise, Antonio Damasio, in his book *Descartes' Error*, tried to persuade us that Descartes's famous saying is incorrect. Damasio states that thinking does not prove existence. The mind is not separate from the brain. The mind is created by the brain through complex physical processes (Damasio, 1994).

A strong force of other great minds, Carl Jung and William James, held differing beliefs and different approaches to the study of the mind. Jung went on to describe a "collective unconscious." With this concept he was able to describe how we are influenced by psychic contents that belong to society, a people, or mankind in general. This view included feelings as well as concepts and ways of looking at things. He was very much intrigued by the feeling function of the person as well as the thinking function. William James viewed mental life as real and not just physical reactions to outside stimuli. James did not endorse dualism but he used the term a dualism of perspective. He believed psychology should be able to describe the connections between physiological states and mental states.

Jung and James used an introspective, reasoning approach to studying the mind but based their approach on experiences with subjects. Unlike their experimental and behavioristic colleagues, they were more impressed by what happened to subjects than what happened in the laboratory. Theirs was an approach that mimicked somewhat the ancient philosophers but was grounded in phenomenological experiences. Of particular importance to us is James's description of the self: "There is a personal self that separates one's consciousness from that of others and that knows, from moment to moment and day to day, that I am the same I was a moment ago, a day, a decade or a lifetime ago. From the beginnings of psychology, thinkers had struggled with the problem of who or what knows that I am I and that my experiences have all happened to the same Me. . . . What substance or entity, what watcher or monitor, accounts for the sense of selfhood and of continuous identity?"

As we know, the classical answer had been the soul, or in more contemporary terms, the transcendental self. Even though the experimental psychologists of the century did not discuss the soul, and the British Associationists laughed it off as a connected chain of passing thoughts, James was able to find a way to restore the concept of self as a meaningful and researchable focus for study. James questioned what accounted for the sense of "me-ness," selfhood, and identity. How was it that we are sure we are who we were a while before? He supported the notion of an empirical self that had several components: the material self, which consisted of the body, clothing, and possessions, the social self or selves, and the spiritual self, which was believed to be the person's inner or subjective being.

Later the humanists like Abraham Maslow and Carl Rogers started describing a self that had other capabilities like self actualization, self esteem, love. Maslow (1908–1970) became the leader of the humanistic psychology movement of the 1950s and 1960s. He described human needs—physiological, safety, social, self-esteem, and self-actualization. Self-actualization is described by Maslow as the need to fulfill oneself, to become everything that one is capable of becoming. Maslow's hierarchy of needs again described the inner self. What is it about man that makes him desire to achieve? Rogers, another humanistic psychologist, describes in many of his works how in a therapeutic relationship the client discovers the self. This discovery involves working through facades and reaching the person that lies underneath. The real self becomes more openly aware of his own feelings and attitudes. He sees that not all trees are green, not all women rejecting. His true self becomes more fully expressed (Rogers, 1961).

PARAPSYCHOLOGY

The soul remained the purview of religious study until parapsychologists attempted to study it scientifically in the late nineteenth century. Parapsychology was heavily influenced by the research traditions of psychology, since many psychologists became interested in parapsychology. Few theories were developed to guide the development of the discipline, which was more research focused. The early research studies of parapsychology are presented in Chapter 9, since the chapters that follow are the extrasensory experiences. However, there is one parapsychologist who theorizes and makes a link between our senses and parapsychology. Peter Sanders (1989) theorizes that there is a psychic reception area in our bodies consisting of psychic feeling, psychic vision, psychic hearing, and psychic intuition. He describes the area in the following way: "All our senses, physical and psychic, function in part by receiving and responding to some form of energy. Physical vision depends on the energy of light waves striking the eye. Physical hearing senses the vibrational energy of sound waves. Taste and smell function through chemical energy reactions between certain molecules and the receptor cells of the tongue and olfactory areas. The psychic senses follow a similar pattern, except that the energies they interact with cannot be discerned physically or measured by current technology" (Sanders, 1989, p. 13). Chapter 9 describes in more detail some of the assumptions and general studies carried out by parapsychologists.

PHYSICS

Until the nineteenth century physicists using Newtonian mechanics described the universe as a huge mechanical system. Newtonian mechanics was considered the ultimate theory of natural phenomena. Soon, however, new physical phenomena were discovered that did not fit the tenets of Newtonian physics (the anomalies described by Thomas Kuhn). In the early twentieth century, Michael Faraday and James Clerk Maxwell described field theory as a more appropriate way to explain these new physical phenomena. The field theorists gave birth to the concept of a universe filled with fields that create forces that interact with each other.

In the 1920s, physicists started describing subatomic particles. Scientists described the energy of heat radiation as not continuous but in discrete energy packets called quanta. Einstein also supported the idea that electromagnetic radiation can appear not only as waves but also in the form of these quanta. These quantum physicists, as they were soon called, established some new principles that they believed governed the activities of these quanta. The uncertainty principle was formulated by Werner Heisenberg in 1927. He stated that the very act of measurement or observation emitted sufficient energy to alter the system that is observed, thus precluding total predictability. This was, of course, contrary to the objectivistic view of science—what is real is what can be observed and studied through our senses. Suddenly there were physicists saying that our act of observing in fact changes the reality of what is being observed.

Another important principle, the principle of complementary, was described by Niels Bohr. Bohr observed atomic interactions from experimental data and noted that electrons appeared to jump from one orbit into a different one without seeming to pass through any intervening space. He stated that sometimes electrons behaved as though they were particles and other times behaved as though they were a wave. Bohr then went on to say that wave and particle theories were complementary to one another. He stated that a photon or electron manifested itself as a wave or particle depending upon the particular experimental measurement. Quantum physics also established the view that position and momentum of an atomic particle are complementary quantities that can only be approximated and not precisely known. Quantum theorists also present the space-time concept in a different way. According to Einstein's theory, time, mass, speed, momentum, and energy may be different for all observers. In fact, the concept of time is dependent upon having an observer. If we were able to place ourselves in a position where we could see everything about the universe, there would be no time. There would only be the universe. However, science as we know it is the study of an object or a phenomenon occurring in a particular set of space-time coordinates. Because quantum physics postulates a unifying principle of complementarity, it helps us understand how a person can be matter and energy that are different from Cartesian dualism. Some quantum physicists contend that consciousness may be controlled by the same processes that govern the behavior of subatomic particles (Pelletier, 1985).

J. K. Arnette elaborates on the relationship between physics and human nature in two articles he wrote on a theory of essence (Arnette, 1992, 1995). This theory is based on the physics of electromagnetism and quantum mechanics. According to Arnette "the body acts as a transformational system for the essence. The body detects electromagnetic auditory, thermal, chemical, and mechanical information and transforms via the peripheral and central nervous systems into an electromagnetic energy pattern in the brain that the essence can sample. The essence is dependent on the accuracy and integrity of physical (biological) systems, both sensory and motor, for the sensory data and physical causality it needs in order to negotiate the world and life in it" (Arnette, 1995, p. 97).

M. Germine (1991), a psychiatrist, hypothesizes the existence of a nonlocal model of consciousness based on quantum physics. Germine believes that the reductionistic, derterministic attempts of neurobiology have failed to produce a definite seat of consciousness. He proposes that consciousness is not localized in one area but rather generalized mental events. In his description, Germine describes the conscious "I" as initially observing brain states. This act of observing then has a role in shaping these brain states in a manner consistent with Heisenberg's uncertainty principle. "Once the assumption is made that our consciousness observes brain events, the conclusion that consciousness has a role in shaping these events becomes inescapable, since the observer always influences the system being observed. Information is generated as a result of any conscious influence, no matter how minor. In order to account for the information content of consciousness, only a very small influence need occur. The magnitude of the influence is in keeping with the magnitude of quantum processes" (Germine, 1991, p. 282).

To date physicists support the notion that we do not have the capability to totally explain human consciousness. They believe that four fundamental forces account for all known phenomena: gravity, electromagnetic forces, weak and strong nuclear forces, and the possibility of one additional force to account for certain inexplicable phenomena not yet susceptible to detection by instruments.

SUMMARY

The current disciplines study and describe the mind and subsequently consciousness and unconsciousness from their individual perspectives. Reading their perspectives collectively, it becomes clear that the physical science and psychological theories are insufficient to completely explain the workings of the mind. All describe the need for an explanation of another force or energy system. That force could be what is described in parapsychology as psi and/or in physics as the additional force or essence.

The next chapter includes a description of Carol's experience while unconscious. Patients' experiences happen undictated by any one discipline's paradigm. You will see that her experiences and the experiences of the patients described in the subsequent chapters need input from all the disciplines to just begin to understand and explain these phenomena.

4

CAROL'S EXPERIENCE

Carol entered Ken Ring's class on death and dying as one of three people who had experienced near-death. She was an attractive, well dressed, friendly woman in her early fifties. We had been reading about NDEs for class, but this was the first time I had ever met someone who had had such an experience. She, like the other guests, described her near-death event. First she remembered a tremendous rushing sound, reminding her of a tornado or a gusting wind. She was then pulled into a tunnel or funnel-like surrounding, going from a wide area to a narrow one. She said that she wasn't frightened but, instead, felt good. There was nothing painful about the experience. She reported seeing her mother who had died nine years before.

She was told by her mother in her mother's native Hungarian language that she and her father (also deceased) had been waiting for her. Carol felt great happiness and comfort. Her mother took her by the hand. She was surrounded by very beautiful marble and wonderful music. She saw her father and others whom she did not know. The entire space was totally filled with light and she felt it surrounding her. The whole experience was very peaceful.

Suddenly, this environment was gone, and Carol could again feel tremendous pain. She remembered reaching a point at which she knew she had to come back but wasn't sure how that happened.

I was fascinated by Carol's experience as well as those of the others. Carol also talked about what she heard while doctors and nurses discussed her when they thought she was unconscious. I can still remember thinking, "Oh, my God, she remembers what it was like when she was unconscious." I listened to every word. I later interviewed Carol for more details about her experience.

At the time of her unconscious experience, Carol was a 47–year-old married woman with a history of hypertension. The unconscious episode occurred when she was at home alone and began having chest pain. The pain increased in severity until she became unconscious. Three days later her son found her, still unconscious. She was rushed to the hospital, admitted to the intensive care unit, and placed on a respirator. She was in the intensive care unit for approximately two weeks with a diagnosis of cardiac arrest and a questionable cerebral vascular accident.

"I remembered hearing my minister and doctor call my name. When I looked up and saw the two of them standing there, I thought I was at my funeral. I kind of chuckled. I didn't know you could see at your funeral. I was supposed to be dead and how come I was able to see? I laughed and chuckled about it. It was brief and it was gone.

"The next thing I remember was my children. I remember my one son calling me. 'Mom, Mom,' he kept saying. 'If you can hear me move your toe.' I thought that was funny. I tried to move my toe. It was taking work. I was mentally bringing action down to my toe. I remember hearing him and trying with all my might to move. Later I heard my other son say I know you want to live. That was when I realized I was still alive. My daughter said 'Mommy, I know you want to live. We need you more than we ever did. I know you want to live, I see you fighting.' But then I was gone again."

"When you say gone again . . .?"

"I would go into unconsciousness. It wasn't just nothing. It was a dark, dark, warm place. It didn't frighten me—but it was always very dark—just darkness and warmth."

"What other conversations did you hear?"

"After that I don't remember my children. I don't remember my husband except for one experience. I knew he was there. I could hear him asking a lot of questions. I could hear him—he had a very harsh voice—a loud voice. I was thinking, why is he talking so loud? Then everything seemed very harsh to me—noises were loud and harsh. There were two doctors there, and he was asking a million questions. After he left one of the doctors said, 'Thank God he's gone.' The other said, 'Well, he's kind of a loyal guy, isn't he?' The first one said, 'Yes, but what a pain in the butt.' I could hear myself chuckling. Gee, they really nabbed him, that's my husband—loyal as hell. It'll kill him but he'll be there. He was always very angry with me. I had a lot of back surgery before and he would come in and shout at me. I remember a couple of times that they refused to let him visit me because he used to upset me so badly. When he visited me, I could sense his anger and hostility and it frustrated me. I just kept going back into this dark, dark place.

"After the doctors said this about my husband, they started talking about me. 'There is nothing on the left side,' one said. 'She'll probably be a vegetable. I doubt, I can't believe this woman's going to make it,' the other responded. I remember saying, 'What the hell's going on here?' I got very agitated. I started trying to move around. The next thing I knew they knocked me out and I was in the darkness again."

"What was the significance of their comments for you?"

"Frightened the hell out of me. It frightened me and made me feel hopeless. Really feel hopeless—like there's nothing. I wasn't afraid to die. I had died. I knew I had died. But my awareness was here. I knew what it meant here, where I was."

"Do you remember anything else?"

"One day my regular doctor came in. He sat on the chair near my bed. He was a good friend besides being my doctor. I could tell he was upset at the way I was. He looked like he was crying. He didn't know I was conscious. At that moment, I was able to get out of my physical body. I put my arm around him and told him I couldn't bear to live. I couldn't bear to live. I'm tired and I can't fight anymore. Then plunk, I was back in my own body. I knew somehow I had communicated with him but it was an out-of-body experience at that point."

"What did you think of that experience?"

"About five months ago, I told him about this experience. He said, 'Hell, no.' I said, 'Hell, yes. I could even describe what you were wearing.' He said that no one was sure what was going to happen. They never expected me to live."

"Were you aware of anything else going on?"

"I also knew there was a love affair or a thing going on between one of the nurses and one of the doctors. It was like I could read their minds. I could feel the emotion. It was so spooky. I would chuckle to myself and it cracked me up—this young doctor and young nurse. I thought it was so funny."

"What kind of thing could you sense?"

"I could sense that there was a great awareness between them. I could feel the love. There was a tremendous emotion involved. During that period I can also remember the aides coming in to clean the floors and some of the nurses. One nurse would come in and never talk to me. She washed and turned me like I was a log. She was cold, unfeeling. I had another nurse that was wonderful. One day I remember I could feel someone touching me. This nurse, Mary, I called her, was washing my face, taking my blood pressure and pulse. I could smell that I had soiled myself. I could feel her pulling down the covers and knew she was starting to change me. Another nurse came over and asked Mary to go to coffee with her. Mary said, 'No, I can't leave her like this. She's my patient, and I'm going to change her now.' At that point I started to cry. I felt her love.

"She said, 'Rest, Carol, don't be frightened. I can see you are frightened. You're so much better.' At that moment I knew I was going to live, I was going to live. I felt her response to me. Like my brain was intact. I could hear. I didn't know if I could talk. I heard them say, 'We don't know if she'll be able to talk, we don't know.' A doctor came over and said, 'I think this woman is going to be fine. I think she's going to make it. I can always recognize that look. She has that look, but she's very frightened right now.' I remember this doctor very well. He used to come to me and he would talk and talk and I felt very comforted. I think he was looking for responses from me. Eventually I got so I could shake my head.

"Then things started happening. I was having dreams. It was the strangest damn thing because in my dreams all the nurses who were taking care of me took part in the dream. I was in a big long hospital room but my bed was the only bed. When I think about it—the bed—it was like an old fashioned iron bed painted white. I was in a bed like that but I was tied. My wrists were tied. I was in a ward. There were windows on this side and the other side but it was just before darkness and all I could see was one light bulb way at the other end and that's all I could see—everything seemed very dreary and dark. I remember thinking why am I alone in this big room. The windows have no curtains or drapes. I didn't know where the hell I was. It was cold. It felt very scary and all of a sudden I could hear this rapping on the window right behind me. I tried to turn and it kept going and it got louder and louder and louder. It was like scratching but on glass. You know that terrible sound and I was getting terrified—so terrified—and then it would stop and then I would quiet down, and then it would start. My head was ice cold and sweaty. I could feel myself soaking wet, covered with perspiration. I was in just incredible blind terror. I didn't know where I was. I questioned the possibility of being in another reality. In my whole life I never went through something like that. The terror was overwhelming. Then all of a sudden this blond nurse comes in. She was big busted but looked very kind. I begged her to untie me. Please untie me. She said she couldn't untie me because he doesn't want me to. Please, I pleaded. All right, but, I have to give you something to quiet you down. She gave me a shot in the arm. And quietly I was gone again.

"The next thing I remember I was awake. I was on a cot but it was on a big porch that looked out over a big hill. I'm still, but I

see the blond nurse and another nurse that reminds me of a movie
star—a tall, elegant lady with her hair up in a twist . She had a long
medical coat. Six nurses are all around me. The blond, very com-
passionate looking. There was one, the intellectual, intelligent,
competent one. The other one was kind of cold. The little nurse was
very efficient, very effective. One had a spiritual, kind of arty look.
She was a dancer, I knew she was a dancer. But these two
appeared to me. Later I realized these were all parts of my own
personality. Each of these nurses who were in reality me. I
remember seeing them but somehow in my mind these were parts
of my personality.

"The next thing I remember—suddenly I was in a large room. It
was a room in a house my son and I had looked at. It was one big
beautiful room with polished oak floors. It had a stage and chiffon
curtains, and I'm in that room alone. All of a sudden comes this
man who was this doctor that was taking care of me with the half
glasses. He had on a trench coat and a hat like Colombo style. He
jumps down off the stage and comes up to me. I said to him, 'You're
the one that is behind all this. You're the one that's causing me all
the suffering—all the agony.' But this is the doctor with the half
glasses, and I said, 'Why are you doing this to me?' All of a sudden
he was down on his knees. I looked down on him and my first
impulse was to hit him. I looked down at him and got down and put
my arms around him. I said, 'I know who you are—you're Mephistopheles.' I didn't know who the hell Mephistopheles was. I never
read of Mephistopheles before. It must have been something I heard
of. I realized who he was, that he represented evil, and all my life
I grew up questioning what is good? What is evil? What is right?
What is wrong? Later I learned Mephistopheles was the devil in
Faust.

"'I understand who you are and I understand why you are the
way you are,' I said. I put my arms around him and he sobbed, and
all the women around me came over and said, 'OK, you can go
now. We're not going to keep you any longer.' All of a sudden the
fear was gone, the terror was gone. I remember the nurse coming
over and saying, 'She's awake. She's fully alert.' After that I

remember I was mostly awake. I remember my brother and his wife coming in, and my children. I started getting better the moment that nurse Mary took care of me. I was in and out, but from then to this last experience I was gradually getting better.

This experience also carried over to my personal life. Months later my husband was beating me and I looked at him and said, 'You are Mephistopheles,' I told him. I realized how I had been trying to overcome being frightened of him, and that dream or whatever it was helped me do it."

Carol later talked with the psychiatrist who had been counseling her and her husband. He was amazed at the level of understanding she had come to while she was supposedly unconscious and so close to dying. At the time of my interview with Carol she was happily divorced and had completely recovered from any physical infirmities.

The many states of unconsciousness Carol experienced are described in detail in the subsequent chapters. Carol experienced unconsciousness, inner awareness, perceived unconsciousness, near-death experience, and two types of extrasensory experiences: five of the five states described by patients from the research, although she did not experience all the components or substates. In the following chapters, each state and substate will be described by examples from the subjects. Relevant research and explanations will also be reported.

5

TOTAL UNCONSCIOUSNESS

Several patients in this study reported experiencing nothing during the time they were unconscious. They remembered what they were doing immediately before they passed out and then waking up. One difficulty that occurred in deciding how many patients really experienced nothing is the discrepancy between the subjects' determination of unconsciousness based on their awareness and the caregivers' observations. In some cases, the subjects' determination of when they were unconscious was different from the caregivers' determination (Figure 5.1). I would ask the subjects during the interview what was the last thing they remembered before becoming unconscious. It was not unusual for a subject to describe what she or he had heard during a cardiac arrest. Since they were aware, they rightfully described themselves as conscious. However, since their eyes were often shut and they were not talking or moving, the caregivers thought they were unconscious.

The experiences reported and discussed in this chapter are those of the patients who did not remember any occurrences during the time

Figure 5.1
Comparison of Patients' and Caregivers' Perception of
Awareness

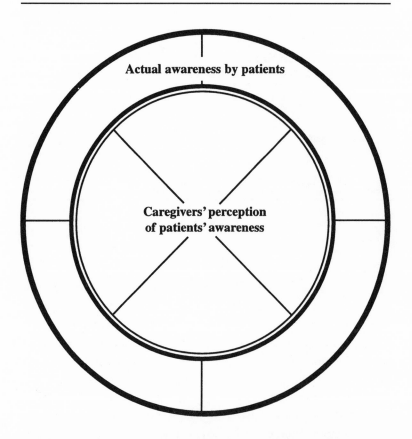

the staff thought they were unconscious. They fit the definition of unconsciousness put forth by Fred Plum and Jerome Posner (1982). "Consciousness is the state of awareness of the self and the environment and coma is its opposite, i.e., the total absence of awareness of self and environment even when the subject is externally stimulated" (Plum and Posner, 1982, p. 1). Total unconsciousness, however, is not without its subtle differences in the type of experiences that patients have had. Some had warnings of an unconscious episode, some had brief experiences, some longer ones. Some also lost memory for events immediately preceding the experiences. Reactions to being unconscious also depended upon the personality of the individual and the type of the experience he or she had.

BRIEF UNCONSCIOUS EXPERIENCES WITH AND WITHOUT WARNINGS

In most cases the subjects who experienced nothing remembered what they were doing immediately before they passed out and then waking up. Some subjects had very brief episodes of unconsciousness, while with others it was more extensive. The subjects who had chronic illnesses often experienced a warning that unconsciousness was imminent. This was not true with patients who became unconscious because of accidents. The following case is that of a 68–year-old woman named Claire with severe cardiac arrhythmias; she had several brief episodes of unconsciousness. In this subject's case, the husband was present and also described what she looked like while unconscious.

Claire

"What was the last thing you remember before you became unconscious?"

"The first time I was sitting at the kitchen table reading the paper. The next thing I knew, I said to my husband that I felt awful. Don grabbed me and sort of shook me and I came out of it. The next time it happened I was in bed. I was asleep."

Don said, "I can tell you she was making some of the weirdest noises you ever heard in your life. It was sort of a choking. That's what woke me up. That particular time her eyes were rolled back. I wasn't sure she was breathing. I had some CPR training and started to give her CPR. I think I gave her three or four breaths when she started to breathe again."

Claire continued, "Another time was about a week ago in the evening. I was sitting in a chair in the kitchen and all of a sudden I said, 'Oh, I feel awful,' and he grabbed me. I came to right away, just like that."

"When you said you felt awful, what was that like?"

"Like I'm blacking out. I feel a wave coming on. I just feel awful."

"When you black out, do you have any recollection at all about that experience?"

"Not a thing. It's just that all of a sudden I'm aware that either Don or somebody is working over me."

"When you start coming out, how does it feel?"

"I'm wide awake each time, aren't I, Don?" she asked.

"I don't know how you feel," he replied,"but you look as though it's like a curtain was lifted. It's not a slow process of coming out, it almost happens in seconds."

Rebecca

The following case is a young woman, Rebecca, who became unconscious because of a brief diabetic episode.

"I had been sick with a virus and I was getting weaker and weaker. My boyfriend came to pick me up for a dance and I was just lying down on the sofa. He asked me what was wrong and I told him I had been sick all day from a virus. He asked what he could do, and I said just keep getting me some juices and water and call the doctor when you have a chance to. That was the last thing I remember."

"Did you slip into it or was it a sudden experience?"

"It actually happened over a period of several hours. I felt very sick to my stomach at work and by the time I got home I was sick."

"So the last thing you remember is telling him to get you some juices and to call the doctor?"

"Right."

"Then what do you remember happened?"

"My boyfriend told me he wrapped me up in a blanket and brought me up to the emergency room. He was worried since I was not able to respond to him, and he said my breathing was shallow. I don't remember him bringing me in."

"What do you remember next?"

"When I woke up and I had all these tubes coming out of me with the intravenous and all that, and I looked up and there was a nurse looking at me. She asked me how I was feeling. She said they were giving me insulin because my blood sugar had risen pretty high—over 700."

"Did you have any feelings when you were unconscious?"

"No, I was completely out of it."

Robert

In the next incident, the subject was a 59–year-old man, injured in an accident while riding his bicycle. His experience is an example of a brief unconscious episode caused by a head injury. Accident patients usually don't experience a warning episode. In the case of head injuries, there is also a loss of memory for the events immediately preceding the event. This loss of memory was not found in patients with unconsciousness associated with a chronic illness. Robert told me:

"I was riding my bicycle when I saw a road coming in from the right side. I looked back and saw two cars coming and let them go by. I looked back and there was no car coming. I put out my right hand as I usually do and moved to my right. The next thing I hear is a horn blowing. The next thing I knew I felt something close to me on my side. Then the next thing I remember I was on the ground and people were around me. I woke up and had some pain. There were people around talking to me, telling me the ambulance was coming."

"Can you go back to when you felt something near you? What do you remember?"

"It was just like things closing in on me. It was all of a sudden I was put into a very small space. I didn't feel any impact. I don't remember any pain. All I remember is the horn, then there was something there that closed in on me, and the next thing I know was that I was on the ground."

Recurrent Brief Episodes

A few patients had recurrent brief episodes of unconsciousness. One man had been bitten by a snake and while he was walking to get help would pass out and then revive himself. Generally patients with this experience did not know how long they were out nor what happened when they were unconscious. As one patient put it, "It's like missing some episodes on a soap opera. You want to be filled in on the events you missed."

While most patients who experienced total unconsciousness had short episodes, there were some patients who were unconscious for long periods with no recollection.

LONGER EPISODES OF UNCONSCIOUSNESS

Patients that were unconscious for a longer period of time added other dimensions to the experience. Most of the subjects wanted to know what was done to them while they were unconscious. If patients were mistrustful or if no trusted family members were with them, they were often scared that something had been done to them that was not in their best interest. Often the caregiver would try to help the patient by reassuring him or her when, in fact, the patient wanted information about what happened.

Agnes

I had spoken to 53–year-old Agnes after she had recovered from a cardiac arrest that she suffered in the emergency room of the hospital. I asked her, "Can you give me a little background that led up to your coming to the emergency room?"

"I didn't feel good. I woke up at four in the morning and had a stuffiness in my middle. I had a problem once before, and the doctor said it was my gall bladder, so I thought it was that. I got up and took some Mylanta, and then I went and opened the door to get some air, but I didn't get any relief. I came back and called my son and told him I was sick and had to go to the hospital. When I got to the emergency room, I had to wait like ten or fifteen minutes. I told the nurse I was sick, not hurting, just this feeling in the middle of my chest. I stood up to tell her who I was but I never got the chance."

"Was that when you became unconscious?"

"Yes."

"What was the first thing you remember upon waking up?"

"I was throwing up so terrible, and they were asking me did I know where I was . . . and what month it was and what day. After the throwing up, I was kind of nervous, because I kept wondering what happened. No one said to me, 'You passed,' or 'something went wrong.' I asked the nurse what time it was, and I was thinking I had something to do that day. I heard someone say, 'It's a good thing she got here just in time.' Then I heard them say something about being admitted, but I wanted to say, 'No, I'm not going to be admitted.' I mean, why? No one had told me what happened."

'What were you thinking then?'

'It was like, 'I'm here throwing up, and my husband is out of town, and my son is out there, and he doesn't know that much about what to do. What is going on?' But I was throwing up so much I didn't ask them. and I was wondering how they got my clothes off me."

"You don't remember that?"

"I don't remember anything. I woke up after passing out, and someone had taken my clothes off. All I could think about was what was going on. I'm seeing these people and the nurse is telling me it's going to be okay. Why is she telling me this? It was scary."

As you can see, Agnes's lack of knowledge was frightening and disorienting. The fright can be particularly strong if the emotionally significant person isn't with the patient. Since Agnes's husband was someone she trusted and depended upon, not having him there increased her feeling of vulnerability.

One patient had been unconscious for more than two months and had no memory of any experience during that time. His family had visited him daily and of course he was subjected to all the treatments associated with a hospitalization, yet he had no recollection of any events. When I talked with him about his experience he was clearly disappointed that he couldn't remember anything. He wasn't concerned about what had been done to him, however. He had heard about near-death experiences and the like and wanted to know why none of these experiences had happened to him.

In Pamela's case, she had an unconscious episode because of a car accident. This incident provides an example of how the component parts come together to form a complete experience for the subject.

Pamela

Twenty-eight-year-old Pamela was hospitalized following a single-car accident. I began our discussion by asking her, "What was the last thing you remember before you became unconscious?"

"I remember driving my car but not being sleepy. But I was, I guess. It was raining. I had had a fight with my boyfriend. We had gone out to dinner and had a couple of glasses of wine. I was supposed to sleep over at his place, but I decided, 'This is it. I'm not spending the night here.' So I got in my car and drove home. I shouldn't have. I was too tired to be on the road. It was late, I had a couple of glasses of wine—a couple of glasses in me is a lot. I was emotionally upset."

"What happened while you were driving home?"

"I must have fallen asleep. Suddenly, I woke up and saw a stop sign. I slammed the brakes on and lost control of the car. It hit an island in the middle of the road. That was the last thing I remember before the paramedics came."

"And then what happened?"

"They strapped me down, and I freak out when I get strapped. I can't be restrained. They had a thing across my chin, and I remember saying, 'Don't do this to me.' My sister, when I was younger, used to sit on my legs in bed and hold me down and put a pillow over my face. I just developed a fear. I remember feeling that I couldn't live in this restraining position and them telling me,

'Pamela, we have to do this because you may have broken bones.' But that's all I remember of the accident. It's just a blip."

"After the paramedics strapped you down, what is your next recollection?"

"Being in the hospital . . . having them take blood from me. And going for a CAT scan. Everyone was sticking needles into me . . . running around in the Emergency Room."

"Do you remember what triggered your awareness?"

"Probably a needle. I remember telling them that my head really hurt. They were drawing blood, and I was telling them that I needed something for my head. Then, I was going into the CAT scan. I remember the machine and asked somebody what it was, and they said it was the CAT scan because I banged my head really hard. I don't remember being inside the machine."

"What happened after the CAT scan?"

"Someone was telling me that we have to take you to another hospital because you have a head injury, and we don't have a neurological unit. Then I woke up in the ICU in the morning with my parents there and Carl, my boyfriend. I remember waking up in lots of pain because of the catheter in me."

"What kind of catheter?"

"For urine. That was the most painful part of the hospital experience. I don't have much recollection of anything in the hospital, but I remember that. The people were kind of vague."

"What do you mean?"

"I never saw nurses. It seemed like they just kept drugging me and drugging me. No one came to help me walk around. The doctor said he wasn't going to release me until I got out of bed and proved that I could stand up and walk. But I couldn't if the nurses wouldn't come and help me get up and get around. I kept saying, 'When am I going home?' And they kept saying, ' Have you walked yet?' But the nurses kept drugging me."

"What did the doctor say to this?"

"I told him that I wasn't going to ever get well just lying in the bed like this, and I finally convinced them to let me take a shower. I walked to the shower and took a shower, and the next day they let me go home. I remember feeling very confused and dizzy . . . and I lost a lot of memory."

"Could you expand on that a little?"

"I used to have an extremely keen memory and didn't have to write things down. I could go to the grocery store and do all my shopping and not forget little odd things. But I lost all that. Just today, I had to drop something off to a client and I forgot it on my desk. I had to drive all the way back to the office and then back to the client's house . . . which is not like me at all. I feel a lot different. My brain has definitely changed since the accident. My neurosurgeon told me that it might take eight months to a year to get everything back. I was out of work for three and a half weeks, but I had to go back financially. I told my boss I had a problem—I had a pretty intense job at the bank at the time—and he just told me, 'Come in when you want, go home when you want.' If it wasn't for him, I probably would have lost my job."

"How was it at work?"

"I had to go through all my computer stuff and my mail and reread memos to get caught up on all the projects I had. I warned everybody that I wasn't an asset to them—more like a liability. Everybody was real good about it. When I was home—before I went back to work—I just got some inner strength to do the things I normally wouldn't have done—like change careers."

"When you say 'inner strength' what do you mean?"

"I have a totally different outlook on life. I felt like I was given a second chance at life. I mean, my car was totalled. It rolled twice across sixty-six. The roof was crushed on the passenger's side, and the only thing that kept it up on my side was my head. So I feel like someone is telling me something. I was so unhappy before the accident about the way my career was going, but I didn't have the courage to take the plunge and change. When I was home—after the hospital—I didn't want to go back to the bank. Usually I'm climbing the walls without work to do, but this time, I didn't want to go back. I wanted to work, but not at the bank."

"How is that going?"

"I'm not as focused as I used to be. I feel like my brain is all over the place. Jumbled. Right after the accident I had to have people say things two or three times. I remember going back to work and looking at my computer terminal and having to read things three or four times . . . like a first grader."

"Has that gone away?"

"Yes. But I remember that. I felt disconnected . . . like my mind was separate from my body."

"How did you feel emotionally?"

"Alone. Even with people around me, I felt extremely alone because nobody could relate to what I felt. So I felt different. Alienated. I couldn't verbalize it well enough, like I can now. I couldn't communicate, so I just kind of withdrew. Then, I started to talk about it more and more as I got well."

Pamela was in and out of unconsciousness, and during this time, she asked not to be restrained, she complained about her head hurting, asked for information about the procedures, complained about pain from a Foley catheter, asked for someone to help her walk, and sought help to restore her memory and other mental functions. In Pamela's case, she got explanations of what was happening to her. As mentioned earlier, some patients asked for explanations and received reassurances. Pamela knew from the caregivers what was happening during the entire episode, but she was emotionally and mentally processing the experience differently from the caregivers and her friends and family. The paramedics at the scene of the accident were focused on preventing any extension of a possible spinal cord injury or fractures by restraining her, but for Pamela this experience brought back a frightening childhood memory. Even though the rationale for restraining her was given, no one addressed her rather severe fright. The disconnect between the caregivers and Pamela widened as her hospital experience progressed. The focus of the caregivers was to save her life and prevent further injury, while she was focusing on returning to the state of physical comfort she normally experienced and mentally functioning the way she once did. Particularly difficult for her was regaining her memory and cognitive functions. Most patients who had become unconscious because of head injuries would have been classified as recovered from their accident, and yet many complained of the inability to function at the level of performance they once had. One woman and her husband broke into tears in my office, while discussing the wife, who had brilliant intellectual abilities before her accident and only moderate to good functions now.

We in the medical profession seem satisfied that we "saved a life," but that person has a difficult transition. These patients described marked changes in self-image and also major job changes. They also felt that there were few resources available to help them. From their perspectives, it is not sufficient to have been potential executive material but now function at a much lower intellectual level. They are often dismissed as being ungrateful since their life was saved.

THE RELATED LITERATURE

There were very few studies in the literature that described the incidence of total unconsciousness. Nathan Schnaper (1975), in an early study of 68 patients who had recovered from posttraumatic coma, found that 43 (63%) of the patients remembered nothing about their unconscious experience. Paula Tosch (1988), in a more recent replication of Schnaper's study, found that 7 out of 15 (48%) of her subjects reported no recollection of being comatose.

In the present study, only 27 percent of the 100 patients reported no recollections of their experience, roughly half that reported in the previous two studies. The discrepancy of the incidence of total unconsciousness between the previous two studies and this one could be due to a larger sample size and documentation of the difference between the time the patients said they were unconscious and the caregivers' determination of the state. If the subjects in this study told me that they heard what was being said and were perceived to be unconscious by the caregivers, I classified them as experiencing a state called perceived unconsciousness. This state was not described in the other studies. That state accounted for 27 percent of the patients and is discussed in the next chapter. I think it is more accurate to estimate that only one in four previously unconscious patients will have no recollection of any experiences during the time they appear to be unconscious.

There were several patients in this study, Robert and Pamela being the two described in this chapter, who became unconscious because of head injuries. The unconsciousness experienced by these patients can be explained by the current known physiology of the brain. As was described in Chapter 3, there is considerable agreement that the reticular formation regulates consciousness— the ability to be aware. The integration of the reticular formation with the cerebral cortex enables us not only to be aware but also to understand what is happening in our environment. Damage to the brain can alter a person's consciousness, either through direct external trauma or swelling or bleeding leading to increased intracranial pressure. Severe trauma can obviously lead to some permanent damage, as in Pamela's case. She did mention, however, some improvement in her abilities. It is not clear how this happened. Since brain damage is expected to be permanent, it is not clear how someone can get better from brain damage. A suspicion is that other parts of the brain take over those functions. How, under what circumstances, and when that happens are not clear.

Less understood also is the retrograde amnesia described by patients with head injury. All the patients in this study experienced loss of memory from thirty minutes to twelve hours before the unconscious episode. Patients who had suffered severe dysrhythmias or cardiac arrests, like Claire and Agnes, suffer temporary imbalances in their circulation and subsequent oxygen levels. If the oxygen level is not diminished too severely or for too long a time, recovery is expected to occur completely.

The diabetic coma Rebecca experienced also was consistent with what we know about the need for glucose to nourish the brain. If there is an excessive amount (since normal is around 100, Rebecca's reading of 700 would certainly be considered excessive), unconsciousness usually occurs.

All the patients in this study who experienced total unconsciousness fell within the known explanation of unconsciousness. However, they were only 27 percent of the total group. The remainder of the patients (73%), even though their unconsciousness was caused by similar pathology, had additional events happen to them. In the next chapter, patients who were perceived to be unconscious and affected by similar circumstances, reported also hearing, understanding, and emotionally responding to their environment.

6

PERCEIVED UNCONSCIOUSNESS

To those around him, a person who is unresponsive to verbal or physical stimuli is perceived to be totally unconscious. Perception, however, is not reality. At some time during his unconscious episode, he (or she) is actually experiencing internal and/or external awareness.

In this study, several patients (27%) heard, understood, and responded emotionally at some time to what was being said while they were presumed to be unconscious but were unable to respond physically or to speak.

AUDITORY CONSCIOUSNESS

Patients often reported hearing sounds around them just as they were becoming unconscious but being unable to respond. These patients said people sounded far away, like they were in a cave. The subjects reported not being able to move or communicate their awareness. Such was the case with Harvey, a 60–year-old man who had a cardiac dysrhythmia at home.

Harvey

"I had been sleeping and I got up to go to the bathroom. I sat on the toilet and suddenly evacuated a huge amount. That's the last thing I remember till I woke up."

"What's the next thing you remember?"

"I had no feelings or anything. I couldn't see. I heard a tramping on the stairs, and then I heard people coming in the bathroom. But I had no sensations. I couldn't see—my eyes wouldn't open. It was very strange. And I could hear the medical technician saying, 'We're losing him.' I tried to say, 'No, you're not,' because I could think and I could hear. But I couldn't move and I couldn't talk—or open my eyes. I was kind of lying there dormant, but I was hearing all the things going on around me."

"What was that like?"

"I had no sensation. I wasn't aware that I was on the floor at that point. I knew I was . . . well, I thought I was alive, but I wasn't sure because I had never had anything like that. I didn't know where I was. Because I couldn't see and I couldn't feel. I could just hear."

I turned to Harvey's wife and asked her what she remembered about that night. "I was aware that he got up and went to the bathroom. I didn't think much about it. Then I heard this terrific thump, and I wondered what it was, and I sat up and looked around. I noticed that the bathroom door was shut, so I figured, well, I'd better check, because it was such a horrible noise. I tried to pick him up, which I managed—he wasn't quite out. Now and then he grunted. I tried to get him to wake up. I let him slide to the floor again, and then I went and called 911 and they came pretty fast, and they got him onto the bed."

"Before they came, what did you notice about Harvey?"

"He was unconscious. He was on the floor, and he didn't move. I went downstairs and opened the door and waited for the ambulance."

"You said that at one time you questioned whether or not he was dead."

"When I was holding him, before I called 911, I was thinking, 'Is he dead?' He had grunted a couple times, but in between he was just a dead weight. His eyes were shut, and I just didn't know."

"Now, Harvey, at this same time, what do you remember?"

"It was very strange. All I could imagine was that maybe I was dead. I didn't know what it's like to be dead, but I thought I could hear but nothing more. No sensation, and I couldn't see. The only thing I recall when I heard him say, 'We are losing him,' was trying to say something like, 'I'm okay . . . I'm not dead or anything.' I think I tried to talk to them, but I couldn't. It was like I had no muscular coordination. I was thinking the words but not saying them. I started to get a little sensation, I think, when they picked me up. Or maybe when they put me on the bed. Then I think I began to be able to speak, and I did say a few things to them."

"Do you remember how it came back to you?"

"I tried to open my eyes, but they wanted to stay closed. The muscles didn't work. I guess the first thing I regained was my voice, because I was able to talk. I don't know if I remember being moved—being lifted onto the bed—or if I just remember being on the bed."

"How did this experience effect you?"

"It was a very relaxing experience, though. I'm not afraid of death. My attitude is that I'm not afraid to die. I sort of look forward to it, kind of like a new experience—a new adventure. So I'm not worried about it, and I was thinking, 'Well, maybe this is it. He says that I am dying.' That's more or less what I interpreted. It didn't trouble me as a concept, it's okay."

TACTILE CONSCIOUSNESS

Some patients reported feeling needle sticks and defibrillator shocks when they were presumed to be unconscious and unable to feel the procedures. Such was the case with Ed, who had a cardiac arrest.

"I just lost consciousness. Everything was black. The next thing I remember I was shocked."

"You felt the shock?"

"Oh, yes."

Another patient described the defibrillator shock as similar to putting his finger in a light socket. Martha was someone who could hear and feel other painful events during her cardiac arrest.

"I remember them rushing into my room. I couldn't talk or move. Someone, I think it was the nurse, banged me on my chest. Then more people came. The next thing I remember was feeling a needle in my groin. I felt that. I could hear them talking about what to do next but then I passed out."

During most incidents of perceived unconsciousness, the patient is aware that she has been "out" for some time. In one unique twist, however, I spoke with Robert, who had gone to the electrophysiological studies (EPS) lab for tests. One nurse who was present during his study had reported that Robert had been unconscious during the test and would be a good candidate for my study. However, Robert said he never passed out but was awake the entire time.

Robert

"Can you describe to me the events that took place in the lab?"

"Well, I remember being wheeled in and I remember the technicians getting me prepped."

"What exactly did they do?"

"They put in an IV and put a couple more of these patches on for monitoring. They also put a catheter in my groin and inserted one in my neck. They were going to determine if I have a problem with the rhythm of my heart, and I think they were supposed to try to induce the problem through electrical impulses. They had an X-ray unit over my chest. All I remember is feeling this tremendous jolt, and apparently, I passed out."

"You don't remember passing out?"

"I don't, no. I remember listening to the conversation between the technicians and the doctors, and I thought things were going fine. Every once in a while, a slight sensation crossed my chest— sort of a brief flash of tightness—and I remember asking what that was. They said it was natural when they were pulsating the heart."

"Stimulating the heart?"

Yes, stimulating the heart. Then, the first thing I knew, there was this tremendous jolt . . . like what you see in the movies when they resuscitate you. This electrical thing. And I said, 'You guys are getting pretty rough now.' One of the nurses said, 'You passed out, but you're all right now. Everything is fine.' I was still feeling these impulses—like a little tightness in my chest—and the nurse said that they were still stimulating my heart. There was nothing to worry about."

"Do you recall—right before you felt the jolt—what you heard them talking about?"

"I think they were reciting some kind of numbers. If anyone asked me, I would swear that I never passed out. As far as I'm concerned, I went through the whole thing awake."

After speaking with Robert, I sought out Wanda, the nurse who had first reported to me that he had been unconscious, to make sure that I had understood her correctly. "Like I told you," she said, "he was out. Basically, we induced the VT (ventricular tachycardia) and he was in VT. I'd estimate a total of about thirty seconds. The defibrillator was charging, and so on. He had passed out fairly quickly. Prior to passing out, his eyes got that foggy look, and he wasn't responding to me. I was calling his name and tapping on his forehead and shaking him. Then, he got that full mouth breathing and had some twitching. His eyes rolled back in his head, and he went out. After he passed out, we cardioverted him and it took a little while for him to come back and reorient himself."

According to Wanda, when Robert did not respond and his eyes rolled back, she assumed he was unconscious. That was the external look that she and the other nurses and technicians associated with unconsciousness. The patients who passed out during the EP studies generally did not remember being defibrillated. They awoke after that occurrence. Robert was exceptional in that regard.

Other patients reported hearing and understanding what was happening in the external environment later during their unconscious experience. One incident was reported to me by a health care professional rather than a patient.

"I'm an x-ray technician. One Friday afternoon they sent me a patient for a series of head x-rays. The man had had a stroke and was on a stretcher completely out. He did not move. There was no response to anything I said or did. After I finished the 11 pictures, the orderly came down to get him. I said something to him like, 'Why do they waste time sending down these zonked out patients?' He just kind of shrugged and took the patient back upstairs. About a week later, my boss called me into the conference room and said a patient wanted to see me. The patient had checked to see who had taken his head x-ray and told me he heard me say he was zonked out. He had heard every word I said."

EMOTIONAL CONSCIOUSNESS

Some patients were aware of their inner emotional state and responded emotionally to what was happening in their external environment. Patients also reported responding to the emotional bond between them and their visitors or caregivers.

Carol, the patient reported in Chapter 4, was able to hear, see, smell, and give meaning to what she heard being said when it was assumed she was unconscious. In this state Carol recognized her children, husband, doctor, ministers, nurses, and even the housekeeping personnel who came close to the bed. She was also able to respond emotionally. Positive emotional energy increased her will to live, while negative vibrations—like those from her angry husband—facilitated a retreat into deeper unconsciousness.

Another patient, Fred, felt the emotions of the visitors from his office. One woman, whom he described as positive and caring, emanated strong, positive energy. He said he could feel her positivism and that gave him strength to get well.

Patients also were aware of their own emotions. One of the strongest emotional stimuli was being referred to as a vegetable. In one instance Carol overheard the doctors say that there was "nothing on the left side" and that she would "probably be a vegetable." Carol said she got very aggravated and tried to move around. Occasionally she was full of despair and hopelessness when she thought of possibly being lame and dependent for the rest of her life.

After recovering, one of the patients told a nurse that he tried so hard to tell his brother he was all right—that he wasn't the vegetable the doctor had said he was—but he couldn't communicate. In another instance, a patient called a nursing unit after she had been discharged to leave a message for a nurse. She said, "Tell the nurse who said I was going to be a vegetable, that I'm not."

Not all the experiences in this state were negative. Rose, who had always been a feisty woman with a good sense of humor, recounted her own experience after becoming seriously ill and unconscious following major abdominal surgery.

Rose

"I remember lying in bed and my husband was sitting next to me. I could hear him but I couldn't move. I was also tied down. He was reading get-well cards. He came to a card my aunt had sent. She and I had never got along—in fact we openly disliked each other. She had sent this sickly, sweet card and my husband was reading it to me. I was getting mad. The more he read the madder I got, but I couldn't talk. Finally, I was able to raise the middle finger of my right hand to gesture what I thought about my aunt's card."

That response was the first time her husband or any of the caregivers recognized that Rose was able to hear and understand what was happening in the environment.

MOTION

Another common occurrence during the perceived unconscious state was an increase in awareness when the subjects were being moved. Movement seemed to be a stimulus that increased awareness. Such was the case with John who had passed out at home at the time of his cardiac arrest.

"I remember being put in the ambulance. From there, the only thing I remember was being picked up two times. They were lifting me up in the bed. I heard nothing and don't remember anything else."

EXPLANATIONS

The most promising approach to understanding how patients can hear, understand, and emotionally respond to their external environment but not be able to move comes from dream research. There are many descriptions of "dream paralysis" or "Rem atonia" in this literature. Some individuals during rapid eye movement (REM) sleep, the normal dream state, but experience a number of physiological changes including body paralysis. Sleep paralysis is commonly described as one of a trio of symptoms associated with narcolepsy. However, studies have indicated that between 26 percent and 39 percent of healthy young adults reported experiencing sleep paralysis (Fukuda, 1993). A person abruptly awoken from REM sleep may have difficulty moving for a few seconds. In this state of paralytic immobilization, the person is awake but cannot move. It is believed by some scientists that this sleep paralysis is controlled by nerve centers in the primitive brain stem (Godwin, 1994). Other postulate that a neurochemical mechanism is responsible for this paralysis and have documented the effectiveness of some medications in reducing sleep paralysis for chronic experience's (Allen and Nutt, 1993). It is possible that some patients as they become unconscious, and others during the unconscious episode, trigger this mechanism inducing paralysis.

Other than anecdotal reports in the lay press, I am aware of no studies of patients who are perceived to be unconscious while hearing what is being said. Arnold Sadwin, a neuropsychiatrist and psychoanalyst, has done extensive work with patients who have had mild head injuries. He believes many do not remember being unconscious when in fact they were and refers to this altered state as dysconsciousness (Sadwin, 1993). Several studies have been done with patients under anesthesia who reported hearing when it was assumed that they were asleep from the anesthesia. The report of one research project also stated that some patients may have been aware of intraoperative events but that these events are not remembered postoperatively. These authors conducted a study with 48 elective surgery patients at the UCLA Health Science Center Hospital. Every patient was presented either preoperatively or intraoperatively with one of two equivalent lists, each composed of 12 different descriptive phrases. Of the 48 patients, 42 professed to be completely amnesic for events that had taken place while anesthetized. Of the remaining six patients, four had a vague recollection of having dreamed during surgery. Two patients accurately reported intraoperative events. One woman, beside remembering hearing the list of descriptive phrases, also heard someone complaining about her weight. The authors could not show that intraoperative events are consciously remembered (Eich, Reeves, and Katz, 1985).

Howard reported an interesting experience that had occurred to a 19–year-old college student. After a surgical procedure, she experienced bouts of depression and senseless eating, a pattern that had been changed through counseling before the surgery. Through hypnotic regression she recalled events in the operating room, events for which in previous probing she had been amnesic. She recalled the surgeon saying, "She is fat, isn't she?" (Howard, 1987).

There were no descriptions that could be found explaining the mechanism by which subjects could hear, understand, and emotionally respond to what was happening in the environment when they could not move. The closest was a description by Guyton of the necessity of oxygen for cardiac muscle contraction. "The hypoxia prevents the muscle fibers and conductive fibers from maintaining normal electrolyte concentration differentials across their membranes, and their excitability may be so affected that the automatic rhythmicity disappears" (Guyton, p. 146). Altered states of consciousness are frequently accompanied by motor abnormalities, among the most sensitive being the motor system which controls eye movement (Troost and Hitchings, 1989).

While Troost and Hitchings describe the abnormal eye movements associated with stupor or coma, they do not describe which of these abnormalities interfere with vision. The implicit assumption they make, which is the assumption most health professionals make, is that even though their eyes may be open, unconscious patients do not see. A few of the subjects in this study, like Carol, did report seeing and being able to accurately interpret what they saw.

Also there were no descriptions of how movement could trigger awareness. Yet it was very clear from the descriptions of the subjects that they were aware yet could not communicate when they were assumed to be unconscious. Many of them reported movement as a trigger for an increase in consciousness.

What is also clear is that the integrity of the person's personality in this state is maintained. The people all kept the same attitudes, likes, and dislikes they had when overtly conscious. They also responded emotionally to events and people in the same way they did before they became unconscious.

Raphael Gimenez, in an article entitled "A Metaphysical Journey in a Comatose State," described his ability to feel emotional vibrations from his wife while in his comatose state caused by an aneurysm. The aneurysm resulted in a massive intraventricular hemorrhage. "My sense of hearing was acute, as was my sense of smell. I could smell things from the surgery room two floors down. As for my hearing, I was able to recognize my wife's steps from down the hall. I was even able to feel the vibrations emanating from people. I do not know how to explain the vibrations, feelings, but I was certainly communicating with my wife through these senses. I felt her heart speaking for her feelings, and I never felt so close to her as while I was comatose. Often I felt she was a saint visiting me, totally inseparable from me. Her soul was speaking to my soul as though it was the ultimate means of communication and the only means left for us to communicate" (Gimenez, 1992, p. 192).

There are some explanations for how patients can feel the emotional energy of others while unconscious. Field theory as described in Chapter 3 provides the scientific underpinnings in the belief of energy transfer from one person to another. This view of man as energy fields has been described in the works of Martha Rogers, Delores Krieger, and Barbara Brennan. All discuss how knowledge of these fields can be used to transfer positive energy that is healing and promotes improved health. Therapeutic touch, which involves the smoothing of energy fields and the transfer of positive energy to clients, has been extensively used and researched in the nursing field.

Renee Haynes (1981) suggests that psychic healing is based on the transfer of an energy not yet understood but similar to the form of energy involved in psychokinesis (movement of physical objects by the mind). Dr. Bernard Grad at McGill University studied one known healer and demonstrated his capacity to heal wounded mice (Glad et al, 1961). Grad also demonstrated that vials of water held in the hands of healers markedly improved the growth of plants. Speculation was that this healing capacity was due to electromagnetic differences in the body of the healers. However, no unusual magnetic fields have so far been able to be detected around healers.

COMMENT

The one message all the subjects who experienced this state sent was how important it was to be treated as a person. They wanted to be talked "to" and not "about." They wanted to be recognized as having an identity rather than being seen merely as an object. The emotional connection they experienced when someone talked to them was seen as contributing to their emotional wellbeing and encouraged them to fight for recovery.

7

INNER AWARENESS

Nine patients in the study reported no awareness of their external environments but an awareness of their inner selves. Their experiences ranged from their being minimally aware of their own feelings, to dreaming, to having internal dialogues.

MINIMUM AWARENESS

In this state, some patients reported only a sense of light or darkness. Always there was freedom from pain or discomfort. The following experience occurred to John, who was admitted to the hospital because of an acute myocardial infarction.

"What was the first thing you remember?"

"I do not know anymore. It was just black. It was dark. Eventually, I passed out and the pain went away. Then I didn't feel the pain any more."

Brian had this episode occur in the electrophysiology lab: " The last thing that I remember is the doctor starting to count and then everything went blank. That was it. Oh, it was white blank. That was it."

Some patients dreamed during their unconscious experience, like 69–year-old Michael, who was dreaming during his cardiac arrest. He had come into the hospital because of an acute myocardial infarction. This episode occurred a few days after his admission.

Michael

"Tell me the last thing you remember before you became unconscious?"

"Well, I was sleeping. So I did not know at all what had happened. I fell asleep around one or two in the morning. When I woke up I think it was about 5:30 in the morning; all these people were around my bed. I remember I had been dreaming about the Nobel prize for the splitting of the gene. I had read about this the previous week, but it was not something that I really kept on my mind all the time. It was not foremost in my mind, because I did not understand it in the first place. I remember it was a very frustrating dream. It seemed to me they were saying the genes were not always arranged in the best way."

"You were dreaming and then woke up and saw these people around you? What was your reaction to seeing them?"

"I was puzzled. They kept asking me if I knew where I was. I didn't know why all the doctors and nurses were there. As far as I knew I was dreaming and just woke up."

During the time Michael had been dreaming he had gone into ventricular tachycardia, had been ventilated and defibrillated. In Michael's case, it is difficult to know at what time he was having the dream and when he was being resuscitated. Other subjects experienced more self dialogue and a transitional place between life and death. Harry, who was 71, had undergone electrophysiology studies and had to be defibrillated twice to convert him back to a normal sinus rhythm.

Harry

"I remember things were going pretty good. I thought I was going to pass the test, you know. Then I guess my heart started to get a little irregular. Suddenly I passed out. I remember I was in a half way in-between place. I didn't even hear them talking. I am in a place I don't like to be."

" How did you feel?"

" It felt awful. I was like suffocating—like I couldn't breathe. It was more my mind than anything else. Like I am in a bad dream, like a nightmare. Like something you can't get out of. You have some types of nightmares and say this has got to be a nightmare. I got to wake up. Sometimes you wake up and you can pull yourself up. I was trying to get my bearings but I couldn't make it. In other words, it was outside of me. My brain was coming back enough that I knew I was in trouble. I couldn't even control where I was. It was like I was half there, you know. Then right away I knew what had happened, then I said to myself that is where I was. I was coming back. I was so alert that I knew that I was coming back."

"Did you have any pain?"

"No, I didn't have any pain. It was just frightening. It was like suffocating. Like not in control. My brain was just enough coming to. In other words, my brain had to be working a little bit to be thinking all this stuff. But not enough so to do anything about it. Not enough to know where I was or anything like that."

Some patients were fearful that death was imminent and engaged in a struggle to hold on to life. Such was the case with Tony during his cardiac arrest.

"I did not have any pain. I did not have shortness of breath. I just knew I had passed out, stopped breathing. The only thing I remember was trying to come back. That was a struggle. I started talking to myself. It was uncomfortable and frightening. I knew I was going to die. 'Oh, my God, I'm going to die' was what I remember thinking to myself."

RELATED LITERATURE

I could not locate any reported descriptions of patients being aware of an inner self while unconscious. However, the experiences of the patients in this study seem to support the belief that there is a mechanism by which we can have an inner dialogue that is separate from the mechanism that enables us to be in contact with our external world. In Chapter 3, there is a description of William James's belief that we have a sense of "me-ness" which provides our sense of continuity which exists even when our ability to be aware of the external world does not function. Also, our ability to communicate with ourselves and think about that communication can still function when our external awareness is no longer operating. M. Germine describes, also in Chapter 3, the "I" that observes the mind and therefore influences it. This "I" seems to remain intact long after the other functions of the brain shut down.

Lucid dreaming was the closest experience and describes our ability to be aware and conduct a dialogue within ourselves when our conscious mind is closed off to external stimuli. Lucid dreaming is a state in which the sleeper becomes alert and conscious that he or she is dreaming. In this state the dreamer takes control over who appears and what is dreamed. According to Malcolm Godwin in his book *The Lucid Dreamer* (1994), one central issue in the study of consciousness is whether there is any essential difference between the experience of being awake or the experience of being lucid and conscious when asleep and dreaming. Typically, in a lucid dream the dreamer consciously recognizes that it is a dream. According to Godwin, the reality of this type of dreaming "is truly uncanny although paradoxically, the dreamer maintains a clear and lucid awareness that it is only a dream . . . you are awake in your own dreams" (p. 22). Similarly, in the state of inner awareness the person is awake and communicating with himself when he is not externally conscious.

What is most curious is why some patients are able to have this inner dialogue and others in the same situation are not. The patients described in this chapter all had to be defibrillated because of a cardiac arrest situation. However, the majority were unconscious because of atrial fibrillation or ventricular tachycardia, much less lethal dysrhythmias than ventricular fibrillation or asystole. It is possible that the body is less affected by circulatory disturbances in these instances. There may have been enough of a physiological shift to render the subjects unconscious to the external world but not enough of an insult to interfere with the mechanism for internal dialogue. It also seems that the mechanism for inner dialogue and dreaming is preserved over the mechanism for external awareness. Whatever happens physiologically, this inner voice and internal communication mechanism can exist even when the external system is not functioning.

Most of the explanations of the existence or lack of existence of the self are logical or theoretical rather than factual. As has been documented in this chapter, whatever the mechanism, the sense of self and the ability to communicate with self still can exist even in a cardiac arrest situation.

8

DISTORTED CONSCIOUSNESS

Fourteen of the one hundred subjects in the Hartford Hospital study and two from the pilot study described distortions in perception, memory, and personality. The perceptual distortions involved hallucinations, illusions, and delusions. The memory distortions involved loss of memory of the times the subjects communicated with their family members and caregivers. There were also some patients who reported marked changes in their personality during this time. While they described perceptual and memory distortions, some also experienced personality changes that were not described previously.

PERCEPTUAL DISTORTIONS: HALLUCINATIONS

Hallucinations are usually defined as sensory perceptions not associated with real external stimuli. Hallucinations can involve false perception of the auditory, visual, olfactory, gustatory, and tactile senses. Two patients reported such false perceptions. The following is an account from Jim, a patient who had had open-heart surgery.

Jim

"It seemed like I was falling asleep, hallucinating. I was seeing things. I didn't know what they were. They were creatures and bamboo trees. It seems like I went back to sleep and yet I wasn't asleep. It seems like I was gallivanting or moving around somewhere."

"Were there other experiences?"

"When I was sitting here I started looking over there and I said, 'Oh, my God, the blood is moving, the blood is moving all over.' I looked out the window and said, 'Look at those birds out there.' Even now I still see birds out there—and red and dark blood on the wall here. I look out the window and I see these birds over there. When I blink my eyes, they are gone. I look back once here and I see blood running down the wall."

Jim was seeing these birds and the blood as I was speaking to him. Although he recognized that the birds and the blood were not really present, he was still distressed by the experience.

Larry

Larry was a 42–year-old man who had been admitted to the hospital because of multiple injuries and a frontal brain contusion sustained in a motorcycle accident. He, too, experienced several hallucinations.

"You became unconscious because of the accident and then what happened to you?"

"I literally lived lives during this period. The first thing I remember was this aide lifting me. He was hurting me and I remember looking at his eyes and they were not friendly eyes. It was like he was using his hand and was pinching me. I started to fight and complain and in my mind because of my complaint, they took him off the situation. I thought I was then taken to a place that was removed from the hospital. A compound. It was woodsy. There was this tall structure and it was very lonely there. I had no idea I was in an accident or anything. I just knew I was hurt and was there. I was restricted—tied down. As things went on, I had all kinds of crazy thoughts and experiences. There was a very large expanse of water filled with flamingos. They were being herded around and used for food. There were fish there also. It was very cold. My daughter was there searching for the fish. I could see through her eyes and see what it was like. I was a bystander—an observer.

"Then I remember thinking we were going to war but I wasn't able to prepare my household because I was tied down. I repeatedly asked my wife to untie me so I could make preparations for this war. She wouldn't do it. I remember getting very angry about all of this. I remember hearing planes overhead and they were on bombing runs."

"When you were having these experiences did they feel real or like dreams?"

"They didn't feel like dreams—closer to reality."

PERCEPTUAL DISTORTIONS: ILLUSIONS

Four patients experienced some type of illusory phenomenon. Harold Kaplan and Benjamin Sadock (1989) defined illusions as a false sensory perception of real external sensory stimuli. Often, the subjects would falsely interpret the sensory stimuli as harmful. For example, patients commonly assumed that they had been captured or held against their will as part of an experiment. Believing these perceptions to be true, they would try to escape by getting out of bed and pulling out their tubes. Richard was a patient who had had open heart surgery. He had several experiences that were disconcerting to him. At the same time, however, he successfully answered the questions from the mental status exam.

Richard

"I never thought I was in a dream. I thought I was in reality. These people were flying around the hospital like they had engines.

Whatever room I was in there was this woman in the corner behind the door. She slept there. Every time I tried to get off the bed she would get mad. She would say, 'If you don't lie down. . . .' She would threaten me. I told my wife. She said, 'Nah. You're not in a room with a woman that is going to threaten you every time you get off the bed.' She was as real as real can be. Every time I made a move she couldn't get to sleep. She finally started crying and carrying on. I said, 'Don't blame me. It's not my fault. I just want to get the hell out of here.'"

"What else happened?"

"A doctor came by and asked me a whole lot of questions. I answered every one of them. I would say they were all general knowledge questions and the doctor was satisfied with the answers I gave him."

"Did anything else happen?"

"This friend of mine, she was not a nurse, but she was taking my temperature and my blood pressure. I don't know why she would take it. She is not the nursing kind."

Although confusing to the family members at the time, some of these situations were later seen as humorous. One of the women who had had extensive surgery was being visited in the ICU by her husband. In an attempt to boost her spirits, he presented a pleasant, upbeat demeanor. His wife, the patient, said she knew why he was smiling so much—that he was having an affair with a nurse and when she recovered she was going to divorce him.

PERCEPTUAL DISTORTIONS: MEMORY

Patients who had had head injuries often experienced retrograde amnesia and reported not remembering their activities from thirty minutes to twelve hours before the accident. Other patients appeared to be conscious and communicative with the staff but then had no recollection of the events. Staff assumed the patient knew what had happened or remembered agreeing to a certain test or procedure. This caused confusion in some instances with family members. That was the situation with Tom, a 53–year-old man who had been admitted to the hospital because of a head injury.

Tom

"What was the last thing you remember that day?"

"I remember coming down to fix the truck. They said I hurt myself when I was finishing the job that I was doing before, but I had thought that I already finished that job. But apparently I didn't. They said I fell off the staging. I don't remember going to the hospital in the ambulance. I do remember getting in the helicopter from the hospital I was in to this one. It wasn't until I got in the helicopter that I was a little more aware. I don't remember being in the other hospital at all."

His wife added, "But you were talking. You were not unconscious. You were talking to us. You gave the nurse my name and telephone number. All the kids came and they all talked to you. You were in pain, terrible pain."

"That to me is a total loss of time. I do remember getting in the helicopter. I remember having them close the doors down. It was like a dream. I didn't know why they were even picking me up. I just thought it was somewhat like a dream or something. I just figured there was no reason I should be there because I didn't do anything."

"So the last thing you remember was you were working and suddenly you were going on this helicopter?"

"Yes, basically. I didn't understand why I was there. I didn't know what was going on."

Other memory distortions occurred when patients were just awakening. Often, patients would report not knowing where they were. In most cases, patients would not be expected to recognize their environment because it was new to them. In a few cases, however, patients awoke in the same familiar environment and could still not identify it at first. *Jamais vu* has been described as a disturbance of memory involving a strong but false feeling of unfamiliarity with a real situation one has experienced (Kaplan and

Sadock, 1989). The following is Michael's experience. He was a 64–year-old diabetic who had recovered from an insulin reaction in his own bedroom and underwent a short-term distortion.

Michael

"I believe the last thing I remember was having difficulty buttoning down an oxford collar. My legs got rubbery. The next thing I remember is looking up and seeing a guy in a blue uniform. He was asking me questions that I thought were ridiculous. What was he doing in my bedroom? Except my bedroom wasn't my bedroom. Everything was where it should be except there wasn't that sense of familiarity. It is the opposite of *déjà vu*. I looked around and there was a picture on the wall and I said, 'Where the hell did that come from?' I learned later it had been there for a year."

Michael said he later found out that his blood sugar had dropped to 20. It only took him about six hours to get back to normal.

PERSONALITY DISTORTION

In some situations, subjects talked with caregivers and family members but exhibited disinhibited behavior, which ordinarily would have been controlled by their sense of social acceptability. In some cases, they uttered profanities or expressed how they really felt about someone. Ordinarily, they would have kept these thoughts to themselves. The patients later did not remember having said or done these things. Family members would often be dismayed and comment on how atypical the behavior was.

Bill

Bill was a 47–year-old man who had fallen at work and hit his head. He experienced a dramatic change in his personality following this event.

"I was on top of the tanker and slipped on the ice. I fell off the truck and hit my head on the pipeline. The next thing I remember was I was in the hospital and they were shaving off my hair. The guy who is the dispatcher saw me fall. He said [afterward that] I was swearing at the ambulance driver. They put me in restraints."

"What happened later?"

"I started to get my personality back. "

"In what way?"

"Being friendly and jovial and stuff like that."

"Anything else you can think of?"

"Only that it took about two and a half months to grow my hair back."

RELATED LITERATURE

It is not surprising that some of these patients experienced a distorted state of consciousness. With the development of intensive care units (ICUs) in the early sixties came frequent reports of psychiatric symptoms (confusion, agitation, and hallucinations) in patients. These psychiatric symptoms are often called syndromes.

These syndromes have been given different names—postsurgery psychiatric syndrome, ICU confusion or psychosis, postoperative delirium, postoperative encephalopathy, and delirium. We know that the estimated prevalence of acute confusion in hospitalized patients has ranged from 5 to 70 percent, depending on the population studied and the criteria used for diagnosis. The occurrence of acute confusion is highest in elderly patients hospitalized for any reason and in patients following cardiac surgery (Neelon, 1990).

The most recent study of open-heart patients reported a decrease in the incidence of delirium from 38 percent to 24 percent in patients who underwent open-heart surgery (Kornfeld et al., 1978). "The reversible, confusional state known as ICU psychosis is usually noted between the third and seventh day after admission to an ICU and generally resolves within 48 hours after discharge from the unit. A lucid period of two to three days usually precedes the onset of ICU psychosis. It is estimated that 12.5 percent to 38 percent of conscious patients admitted to critical care settings experience this phenomenon. The highest incidence of ICU psychosis has been reported in the surgical intensive care unit (SICU), followed by the medical intensive care unit (MICU), and the coronary care unit (CCU) and general medical and surgical wards respectively" (Easton and MacKenzie, 1988).

These patients' experiences tend to be frightening for the subjects and have a general paranoid quality to them. Very common is a feeling of being held captive and being part of an experiment. One study described the illusions of a 56–year-old housewife admitted because of aortic stenosis, secondary to rheumatic heart disease (Abram, 1965). Six days after surgery to replace her aortic valve she experienced a psychotic episode. The following are the words of a nurse describing her behavior. "Patient is evidently experiencing auditory hallucinations—says she hears her daughter's husband paged over the p.a. system, has been smelling strange gas all day."

When the patient was seen by a psychiatrist, she told him she was convinced she would be taken back to the operating room for more surgery. Also she thought the "new machines" had been brought to her room to do her harm (Abram, 1965, pp. 662–663). Another study of open-heart surgery patients found that eight out of twelve subjects had a major psychotic episode (Blacher, 1972). Five had delusions or hallucinations and three loss of memory and confusion. The following are excerpts from patient descriptions.

"A 43–year-old man with an aortic valve replacement reluctantly described how he knew the staff was trying to kill him by putting the suction tube in his nose. At the same time, he knew that this couldn't be true."

"Two weeks after a combined mitral commissurotomy and aortic valve replacement, a 58–year-old woman woke up one morning and announced that she wondered where she was. 'I then realized where I was and felt alive for the first time. I was in a trance since the operation.' This woman had been observed for more than a week and had seemed perfectly alert" (Blacher, 1972, p. 306).

The experiences of patients in the present study were similar to those just described. The explanations for these experiences fall into four categories: predisposing psychological factors, deprivation, biophysiological factors, and pharmacologic agents.

Predisposing Psychological Factors

Most of the psychiatrists who have conducted investigations in this area have advocated explanations that include the severe anxiety experienced by the subjects. All their subjects came close to dying or at least had some risk of dying. If the threat of death was overwhelming, the psychiatrists believed it could contribute to hallucinations and illusionary experiences.

Psychiatric history and personality type are also believed to be contributing factors. Individuals with preoperative psychiatric illnesses have been found to be more prone to development of delirium when hospitalized with a serious illness (Dublin and Field, 1979). Individuals with dominant, aggressive, and self-assured personalities were found to be the most likely to be affected by delirium (Kornfeld, 1978). A history of a psychiatric illness resulted in the subject's being excluded from this present study.

Deprivation

Several studies have been done on the hallucinations that occur when subjects experience either sleep or sensory deprivation (Helton, 1980; Comer, 1967). Since sleep and sensory deprivation are common in ICUs many believe they can be contributing causal factors.

Biophysiological Factors

Individuals who have been addicted to drugs or alcohol have a predisposition to hallucinations, illusions, and delusions when seriously ill. Since many admisions to ICUs are occasioned by accidents where drugs and/or alcohol have been involved, it is not unusual for drug and alcohol users to go through withdrawal while in the ICU. Patients with chronic cardiovascular, metabolic, or respiratory illness are at a higher risk for develping delirium while in the ICU. Physiologic aberrations caused by hemorrhage, septic shock, anoxia, acid-base imbalance, and other serious physiological changes have been documented in persons with ICU psychosis.

Pharmacologic Agents

Fifteen common pharmacologic agents used in ICUs include acute delirium, hallucinations, agitation, paranoia, confusion, or nightmares as potential side effects (Easton and MacKenzie, 1988). With so many potential causes, it is difficult to establish the necessary and sufficient conditions for a psychotic episode to occur in a serious illness. Since these episodes are transitory, emphasis has been on identifying patients at risk and supporting the patient after the experience.

COMMENT

I hope the descriptions of the patients in this chapter help family, friends, and health professionals understand what the patients are going through in this state. A patient who is trying to get out of bed or is pulling out tubes is probably fearful that someone is trying to harm him. The subjects reported being helped by constantly being told where they were and what was happening to them. If the words were spoken by someone they felt cared about them, the explanations were more often heard.

EXTRASENSORY EXPERIENCES

This chapter begins the section of the book that describes extrasensory experiences reported by the subjects. Since these types of events deviate remarkably from experiences described in the previous chapters, this chapter will provide relevant background information.

Some of the patients in this study reported having one or more of four types of experiences commonly referred to as paranormal: out-of-body experiences (OBEs), near-death experiences (NDEs), near-death visits (NDVs), and encounters with the "grim reaper."

THE STUDY OF THE PARANORMAL

In 1869 the London Dialectical Society appointed a committee to begin a study of spiritualism. William Crookes, a well-known British chemist, became involved with the committee as a consultant because of his scientific objectivity; he became the first British scientist to study the existence of the soul and turned out to be the first of many to engage in this quest. In 1882 the Society for

Psychical Research was started, making it the first organization to officially investigate paranormal experiences. Paranormal experiences include instances of telepathy (communication from one mind to another by extrasensory means) , clairvoyance (ability to perceive objects or events not present to the senses), precognition (to know beforehand), and psychokinesis (the ability to move objects or people with the mind).

Parapsychologists started the inquiry into these paranormal experiences by engaging in experimental studies and were not initially very theoretical. Soon unique methods were used to study these experiences, including the detection of the soul. Some of the first funding in psychical research came from individuals who were interested in knowing whether something survives after death. Some researchers took pictures of the soul leaving the body; some weighed dying patients for weight loss after the soul left the body. Others tried to bring spirits back from the dead. While a number of legitimate scientists were pursuing this investigation, there were many frauds in the field that discredited the study of this subject. Even Crookes himself was fooled on a number of occasions.

In the middle of the twentieth century, several substantial endowments to the American Society for Psychical Research enabled other legitimate researchers to continue looking into the paranormal or extrasensory, as it became called. At this time, parapsychologists began descriptive studies of the incidences of these experiences and the characteristics of those who had them.

Parapsychologists soon found that parapsychological phenomena were quite common in the general population. This is contrary to previous beliefs that psychic experiences were limited to a small, select segment of the population, often considered to be suspect. These were people who were sometimes described as charlatans or crazy persons. The current view of psychic experiences is that they are quite normal and, in fact, are probably normally distributed. Some individuals have a great number of psychic experiences, some have none or very few, and the majority of us have some.

Several researchers and, most recently, pollsters have surveyed the population to determine the frequency with which individuals perceive themselves as having extrasensory experiences. The following is a table from a study by Andrew Greeley, published in 1975, of a survey of 1,460 Americans (Greely, 1975).

Type of experience	Occurred once	Occurred often
Contact with the dead	27%	11%
Telepathic experience	58%	30%
Clairvoyance	24%	10%

In a 1990 poll with 1,236 respondents the following data were obtained:

Type of experience	Percent Occurrence
Mental telepathy	25
Déjà vu	56
Contact with ghosts	5
Knowledge of past lives	4

These researchers concluded that extrasensory/paranormal experiences are common in the general population.

Greeley also looked at the characteristics of the people who reported mystical experiences. He found them to be generally better educated, more successful, and less racist. They were rated substantially happier on measures of psychological wellbeing than those who had not had such experiences. Charles Tart, a well known parapsychologist, summoned up the sentiment of most of the researchers when he said, "The extrasensory is not the exclusive province of a few deranged people" (Tart, 1968).

We know that extrasensory phenomena normally occur in stable, well-adjusted adults. The basic question, however, remains: what is the true nature of these experiences? Can a person actually predict the future? Are the dead spirits real?

It has been argued that incidence itself does not make an experience real. Ross stated that *deja vu* experiences were so common they could not be considered paranormal, but are they real? Just because a large number of the population feel they've been in an unfamiliar place before or had the same experience before doesn't prove they actually were there or had those experiences. Soon some parapsychologists realized that they needed to develop theories and frameworks to guide their experimental studies to better answer these research questions.

Extrasensory experiences did not fit the rules, boundaries, and norms of our current beliefs about normal science. Anatomy and physiology textbooks certainly did not contain explanations or mechanisms for out-of-body experiences or telepathic communication. New theoretical assumptions and frameworks were needed. There was, however, limited funding for the development of such frameworks and few have been described. One exception is the work done by Lawrence LeShan. LeShan developed a theory of parapsychology by studying known mediums and mystics.

LeShan believed that the study of the paranormal is much more than just investigations into unusual activity. He believed it to be the study of the very basic nature of man. Our present cultural picture of man is to see him as rational and sensible, made up of flesh and bone and nerve and totally separate from one another. LeShan argued that not all the facts support this view and that parapsychology is the scientific study of "the damned facts," the ones that cannot be explained by rational science. He asked the question, "What is going on between the sensitive and the rest of reality at the moment the paranormal information is acquired?" He describes his theory of clairvoyant reality as a complete metaphysical system, a coherent, organized picture of the-way-the-world-works in this reality. The following are the components of LeShan's theory:

- Individual identity is essentially illusory. Primarily, objects and events are part of a pattern which itself is part of a larger pattern, and so on until all is included in the grand plan and pattern of the universe. Individual events and objects exist, but their individuality is distinctly secondary to their being part of the unity of the pattern.

- Information is known through the knower and object, being part of the same unitary pattern. The senses give only illusory information.

- Time is without divisions, and past, present, and future are illusory. Sequences of action exist, but these happen in an eternal now. It is the time of all-at-once.

- Evil is an illusion, as is good. What is, is and is neither good nor evil, but a part of the eternal, totally harmonious plan of the cosmos which, by its very being, is above good and evil.

- Free will does not exist since what will be is, and the beginning and end of all enfold each other. Decisions cannot be made, as these involve action-in-the-future, and the future is an illusion. One cannot take action but can only participate in the pattern of things.

- Perception cannot be focused, as this involves will, taking action, and action-in-the future, all of which are impossible. Knowledge comes from being in the pattern of things, not from desire to know specific information. Perception cannot be externally blocked since knowledge comes from being part of the All, and nothing can come between knower and known, as they are the same.

- Space cannot prevent energy or information exchange between two individual objects, since their separateness and individuality are secondary to their unity and relatedness.

- Time cannot prevent energy or information exchange between two individual objects, since the divisions into past, present, and future are illusions, and all things occur in the "eternal now." (LeShan, 1974, pp. 86–87)

If these experiences are labeled as hallucinations, illusions, or delusions, they fit into our current paradigm as psychopathology. If they are interpreted as real, they challenge our understanding of normal science. Not all of us function from the paradigm put forth by these scientists. Religious and parapsychological paradigms accept the possibility of these experiences as occurring not as abnormalities but as phenomena consistent with the beliefs of these disciplines. Some clergy, for example, would have less difficulty believing in the near-death experience as a phenomenon that happens as it is described. It is for the most part consistent with their current view of the after-life.

BIOPHYSIOLOGICAL THEORIES

In 1978, the California Museum of Science and Industry produced an exhibit describing the relationship between energy and
survival after death. The exhibit created phenomenal excitement by
introducing some laws of physics as the basis for accepting the
existence of life after death. The exhibit emphasized the belief that
energy is indestructible, that consciousness can exist independent
of the physical body, and that there was evidence that consciousness
continues after death. The exhibitors presented modern physics as
supporting consciousness as waves and fields capable of existing
independent of brain matter. Similar to the discussion of field
theory and quantum physics in Chapter 3, physics supported new
constructs for understanding the nature of man, constructs quite
different from the biomedical model.

Parapsychologists start out with a belief in the possibility of
extrasensory experiences being possible. They conduct numerous
studies on the incidence of experiences that cannot be explained by
normal science. In general, their research has shown that psychi-
cally-gifted individuals are able to have experiences not explainable by our current understanding of how the body works.
Parapsychology, however, has not been well accepted by main-
stream science and research. There are enough pseudo-psychics to
mar their reputation. Thus, the results of their research is often
suspect. They also are chronically underfunded, which deters progress in the development of their discipline.

Currently, extrasensory experiences are observed in patients
who are being cared for by doctors, nurses, and other health
professionals who have been professionally raised in the tradition
of normal science. This has created not only a dilemma but also an
opportunity. We don't know yet whether these extrasensory experiences can be explained sufficiently by our current scientific
paradigm. We do know that these extrasensory experiences are
occurring in patients without psychopathology. The best predictor
of the occurrence of these experiences is coming close to death. In
our exploration of these extrasensory events, we do not know if
normal science, as we understand it, will be able to explain these

experiences. We may, in fact, be on the verge of creating a new paradigm.

We need to be aware of Thomas Kuhn's belief that our paradigms filter information. If new information does not fit our current beliefs, we disregard or invalidate that information. Since the results of parapsychological studies are often inconsistent with paradigms of normal science, the findings are disregarded not on scientific merit but on the basis of rules and norms from a different tradition. The frustration of parapsychologists and the influence of paradigm filtering is well described in the following quotation.

> When I was young, I believed that if people would only read the existing evidence, people in general and scientists in particular would see the validity of these phenomena (extrasensory) and begin studying them. As a psychologist, I have come to realize that people's beliefs are formed in much more complex ways than simply looking at the evidence. We frequently have intense and largely implicit emotional commitment to our beliefs. (Tart, 1968)

Because the paranormal is often defined as a psychic or mental phenomenon outside the range of the normal, people who have these experiences are often labeled as abnormal. Extrasensory is a general term that includes a wide variety of human experiences having a common characteristic that they should not happen. I believe that "extrasensory" rather than "paranormal" leaves the question of the cause of these experiences open and challenges our boundaries of physical reality rather than labelling the subjects. In this book, then, these experiences will be referred to as extrasensory rather than paranormal. In the next four chapters, each of the four types of extrasensory experience reported by patients will be discussed. In the spirit of openness and awareness of our filtering tendencies, research from both parapsychology and normal science will be described.

10

OUT-OF-BODY EXPERIENCES

An out-of-body experience, or OBE, has been described as the sensation that a person's consciousness or center of awareness is at a place different from the physical body. Seven subjects from the pilot study and the Hartford Hospital study had out-of-body experiences not associated with near-death experiences. The OBE included one to four phases: leaving the body, viewing the body and other activities from a space separate from the body, traveling to other sites away from the body, and returning to the body. The following are descriptions from some of the subjects in this study.

LEAVING THE BODY

Of the patients who reported an out-of-body experience, two had only the sensation of leaving their bodies. A 74–year-old woman, Mary, experienced a period of respiratory distress because of a punctured lung.

Mary

"Would you describe the experience you had?"

"Well, I felt like I was rising above the bed. I was just leaving. I felt like I was rising—going up. I don't know what was around me. You know how when you ride—when you go up. It's just like when you push the button and go up. That's how I felt I was going."

"Were you horizontal?"

"Yes, lying down. Just lying down and going up that way."

"Could you tell if you were connected at all to your body? Was there anything underneath you?"

"No, it was too fast to think about what was happening. I think I was so frightened I woke myself up."

John, a 36–year-old patient who had had a respiratory arrest, had an experience similar to Mary's.

John

"I was restrained and had a mouthpiece in my mouth. I felt like I was dead. It was the most fearful time."

"What was frightening?"

"I was totally paralyzed. It felt like I was leaving my body. I felt like I was going through this little mouthpiece—through the hole in my mouth. That was the most fearful thing. I was crying, trying so hard to get through and couldn't. I was just going into the tube and it wasn't working. I tried, I tried. I was slipping and struggling. At that point I felt like I started to float through the tube."

Mary's and John's experiences were similar to many accounts of experiences when individuals have the sensation of leaving the body. First of all, they experienced the sensation of a part of themselves starting to become separate from their bodies. Most often there is some fear associated with this sensation. It is now evident that some subjects only have the experience of feeling like they are leaving their body. Others feel like they have left their bodies and experience the world from a vantage point that is above the ground.

The following incident was reported by a patient's wife. He had told her about the experience but later could not remember having had it or ever talking about it.

Oscar's Wife

"He said to me 'I had the strangest thing happen.' He said, 'I lost my body.' He went into this explanation of how the nurses had told him if he didn't behave himself they were going to put him in a straightjacket. Then everybody went away. He then lost his body. While in that state, he saw the nurses popping popcorn. When the popcorn stopped, they all 'attacked' him and put a tube down his throat. I asked him if he felt pain. He said he felt no pain since he wasn't in his body anymore. He had stopped breathing, which was why they put the tube down his throat."

Another patient during an electrophysiology study, also reported the early stage of an out-of-body experience.

Andrew

"I was supposed to be laying flat on my back, but it seems like I was standing and the nurses and the people were not around me but down below me. I was in the vertical rather than the horizontal. I would blink my eyes and open them and be back to normal but coming and going. That sensation didn't really bother me—but initially it was kind of frightening, but it didn't stay."

"What could you see when you were standing?"

"Well, whatever was around me. Only it was in the wrong position. The lights were not above—they were in front of me."

"Could you see yourself?"

"Yes, I could see my toes. I would look down like I was standing."

"Did you feel like it was you?"

"Yes."

Another subject, a 50–year-old woman, had the following experience during a cardiac arrest.

Eileen

"I was in a twilight zone. I was looking back at a picture I was in. I felt very distant from the picture."

"What did you see?"

"I was dressed in a turtleneck. A white turtleneck with a black jacket."

"What were you doing?"

"I felt like I was taking control. I felt like I lost my power and was examined all the way through."

Other patients who have more extensive out-of-body experiences will have the sensation of leaving their body but also seeing more activities. Ronald was 59 years old when I talked with him in 1991. Our conversation centered on an experience he had had during a stress test.

Ronald

"I was having a stress test, and part of it was bicycle riding. I blacked out, and it was while I was blacked out that I felt as if I had left my body and was looking down. There were three nurses and a doctor in attendance, and I was above them looking down at them and me, lying on the floor. They were trying to resuscitate me. I saw all of that . . . or imagined that I saw it. But I do recall seeing them bending over me on the floor."

"You were watching all their activities?"

"Yes. I saw myself lying on the floor with everybody scurrying around and trying to revive me."

"How did you feel about seeing yourself being revived?"

"It happened so quickly that I didn't feel anything. I thought it was like a dream, and it wasn't until a day or two later that I talked to my wife about it. I also talked to the doctor, but nobody could give me a good explanation of what had occurred other than, 'Gee, that was unusual.' It didn't bother me, and I didn't have any ill effects from it."

"What do you think happened?"

"My interpretation of it later was that I was probably on my way out and they were bringing me back to life and I was watching the whole episode."

"When you were out of your body, did you have any sense of what you were like?"

"No. It happened so quickly. It was just a matter of seeing myself lying there with everyone working on me. The next thing I knew, it was black and dark, and I woke up in the hospital."

Pain can also be a trigger for an OBE in hospitalized patients. The next subject, Heather, had the most detailed OBE experience of all the subjects I interviewed. She also described how pain influenced her experience, during an incident that had occurred 27 years before our conversation, associated with the birth of her eldest son.

Heather

"It was a very long labor. I was exhausted. I told them I wasn't going to do it anymore. I had been in labor from eight in the morning until eight in the evening. It was really intense. I asked the doctor for some medication, but he said no—that I had to help myself. You know, 'You have to work at it.'

"Of course, it never would have happened no matter how hard I worked, because the baby's head couldn't fit through my pelvis. The pain was really severe, and I remember thinking to myself, 'I've got to get out of here.' I mean, I was getting very nervous and the next thing I remember, I was looking down on myself. I was on the ceiling in the corner."

"You were on the ceiling?"

"I was looking down, and saw myself on the bed. It was pink. The room was a golden pink and very, very bright. I was in something pink and soft. I could look down and see my doctor and myself on the bed. He was sitting next to me, holding my hand. The nurse was on the other side, taking my blood pressure. I felt great.

Light, very light. No pain at all. I could see myself and I wasn't frightened any more."

"Were they saying anything?"

"I couldn't hear them until another doctor came in. They started calling me. Like, 'Heather, wake up,' and the nurse had something she was putting on my lips. The doctor kept saying, 'Wake up.' We have to take you out of here, or something like that. I kept thinking that I couldn't go—that I couldn't leave. I could hear but it was muted, like water in your ear. The new doctor examined me, and then they put me on something with wheels. That's the last thing I remember."

"Do you recall going back into your body?"

"No. I just remember staying in the corner."

"When you were looking down on your body, what was your reaction?"

"Not much. I just felt that if I went back, that I would feel the pain again. It was great where I was. I wasn't surprised and I wasn't frightened."

"Did you feel differently?"

"Not really. It was very light and there was no pain. It was silent. Feeling no problems or worries. Kind of like having a couple of glasses of wine."

"What did you look like? The 'you' on the ceiling?"

"Pink. And the room was pink. I thought afterward that maybe I chose pink because it's such a warm, toasty color. I know I was clothed. I had something on. Whatever I was wrapped in was soft and pink and warm. I felt warm."

"Could you sense your arms and legs?"

"No."

"Were you still pregnant?"

"No, maybe not. I didn't feel ungainly at all, and I was really big. Nope. I wasn't pregnant."

"When you looked at your body, what did it look like?"

"It was a lump in the bed with a cover over it. The doctor was sitting beside me, looking at my fingers for some reason. The nurse was on the other side, taking my blood pressure. Then the other doctor came in, and he did another internal examination."

"Did you know who that other doctor was? Did you see him again?"

"No. I didn't know him. He was just a doctor in a white coat."

"Other than the fact that he had a white coat, was there anything else you remember about him? Was he tall or short?"

"He seemed thinner than my doctor. It seemed to me the other doctor was growing a little bald on the top of his head. To tell you the truth, I wasn't really very curious about the whole thing. I was happy up there. I remember the shimmering waves beneath me, and I knew the pain was beneath those waves. I knew that if I went down there, below the waves, the pain would start again. I knew that as surely as I knew anything."

EXPLANATIONS FOR OBEs

There are three categories of explanations for out-of-body experiences: parapsychological, psychological and bio-physiological theories.

Descriptions of out-of-body experiences (OBEs) by psychical researchers began around the turn of the century. Initially this experience was believed to be a rare phenomenon, since only a few gifted psychics and occultists wrote autobiographical accounts of their OBEs. In the 1950s the perspective changed. Sylvan Muldoon, an ordinary citizen, wrote an autobiographical account of an OBE that occurred when he was a teenager. This book was widely read, and many people wrote to Muldoon about their experiences.

According to Scott Rogo, the publication of so many firsthand cases alerted the parapsychologists to the OBE as a much more common experience. Muldoon's book stirred the interest of Robert Crookall, a British geologist. By 1972, Crookall published three case books of 746 firsthand accounts of OBEs. Muldoon and Crookall gave us the first extensive description of OBEs.

The subjects in these books had varied experiences. Some remembered leaving their bodies. Some reported exiting through their heads. Some remembered being attached by a cord to their bodies. Most remembered being able to see their physical bodies.

When asked to describe what they looked like in their OBE form, some said they could not remember, others that they had another body (Crookall, 1972).

Crookall believed there were a number of circumstances under which the natural OBE occurred: exhaustion, illness, near-death states, sleep, hypnogogic states, relaxing, and meditating. Enforced conditions could also induce an OBE, such as drugs, suffocation, physical or emotional shock, hypnosis, and voluntary induction. Crookall claimed that natural OBEs had a higher frequency of phenomenological qualities and better perceptual, mental, and emotional aspects of the experience.

Some of Crookall's subjects reported going through a tunnel, seeing a light. Today, those occurrences would be called near-death experiences (NDEs). These near-death experiences will be described in Chapter 11.

Crookall's work sparked interest in this area, and other psychic researchers soon began investigating these experiences. In 1978, Karlis Osis and Donna McCormick did a survey of out-of-body experiences from the insider's view. They constructed a 96-item OBE questionnaire that included queries about various aspects of the phenomenon. They received 403 usable responses. Most of the respondents said they saw as they normally did with their physical eyes, but some did report being able to see around corners, behind objects, and through walls. Most respondents had out-of-body visions that were like movies, as opposed to other psychic experiences that came in brief snatches like still photos. Some subjects (34%) felt as if they were engulfing objects in their environment or even fusing with them. When asked how they looked while in the OB state, 30 percent reported themselves as having a "second body," 23 percent reported no form at all, and 14 percent described themselves as a ball of energy or light, a point in space.

In 1984, Carlos Alvarado studied the quality differences between enforced and natural OBEs and found there were no significant differences. He also asked subjects to describe themselves while out of their bodies. His study showed that 35 percent said they were without a body, 23 percent with another body similar to their physical body, 13 percent as a cloud, mist, or ball of light, 7 percent had no recollection, and 20 percent said other.

In 1988, Melodie Olson published a study of OBEs of hospitalized patients. Two hundred subjects were interviewed. Thirty-one reported having had an OBE sometime during their life, six during the current hospitalization. Of the thirty-one OBE subjects, twenty-two reported OBEs related to stress, six related to relaxation, and three were unspecified.

PARAPSYCHOLOGICAL THEORIES

Parapsychologists have studied OBEs using spontaneous case reports and experimental laboratory explorations. While researchers initially focused on descriptions and frequencies of OBEs, by the late 1960s research focused on the question "Does something leave the body during the OBE?" This type of research is often called studies of the separation theories.

Much of the research to test the separation theories focused on two general approaches: the visualization of an unknown or distant object while out of the body, and detection of the traveling self. Charles Tart, a noted researcher, reviewed many historical cases. His belief was that there was enough evidence to verify what subjects said they saw while in their OBE state. The early veridical perception studies in the late 1960s and 1970s were done using "gifted subjects." These subjects were individuals who reported frequent OBE experiences that they could induce at will. Robert Monroe, a Virginia businessman who wrote his accounts in his own book, *Journeys Out of the Body*, was a frequent subject for studies done by Charles Tart. Ingo Swann, Alex Tannou, and Bill Harrary were other noted travelers used in these experiments. In the experiments, targets were set at distant or normally nonvisible places and the subjects were asked to describe what the targets were. Some studies with Swann and Tannou (Osis, 1974) were impressive, often reaching statistical significance. Swann, for example, was placed in a specially selected room and was asked during his OBE to look into a box suspended there. He was instructed to sketch and describe what he saw. Independent judges successfully matched the drawings with the objects.

Research with gifted subjects turned up some surprising occurrences. These research projects were based on the assumption that the people would be subjected to the same set of concerns, purposes, and interests out of their body as they were in their bodies. These assumptions often proved to be unfounded. Subjects in the out-of-body state quite frequently became distracted and lost sight of their original intent. Occasionally, they also became disoriented, finding themselves in locations other than the target areas. Harrary, for example, in his experiments was asked to project to another building to view a letter printed on a poster and affixed to a door. Harrary had difficulty reading the letter (partially because of its elaborate and arty design) but was quick to notice a visitor in the room unknown to the primary experimenter.

While there were some interesting significant results from this type of research, there were also some discouraging moments. Two researchers, Susan Blackmore and William Roll, were able to have OBE experiences. They went to predetermined areas and upon return described the scene they observed. What they found, however, was that what they had seen during their OBE was not there in actuality. During one OBE, Roll went to a room in his house and tried to establish the veridicality of his perceptions.

I got into a room in my house and stood in the doorway in my out-of-body form. I was so excited about the clarity of this experience and so frustrated that I could not really check it. But then, fortunately, the moonlight came in through the double doors and cast shadows on the floor. One of these shadows overlapped the rug. The moonlight hit a round table we had in the living room and the shadow fell across the rug in the living room. I told myself, "Now, I could not have known that this shadow would fall exactly this way at this time. So, I'm going to check it." I went down on hands and knees and put my hand to the floor. I measured the shadow as it stuck out from the rug. I felt the oak grain against my palm. It was so realistic. With this precious information, I moved down a hallway where, for some reason or other, I did not walk vertically: I walked slightly at an angle, as if I was on a different floor. I got into the bedroom which was pitch dark. I plunged into my bed, hoping that I would merge with my own body rather than with my wife's, which would have been really confusing! I aroused my body and went back into the sitting room to check the shadow. The sitting room was pitch black. There was no moonlight. Not only was there no moonlight, but the shadow I saw could never fall the way I saw it, either by artificial light or real light. I figured out that this was a mental world. . . .

Before this I was convinced that life would continue for me in the out-of-body form I was familar with in my out-of-body experiences. Now, having done further exploration of one kind or another, I feel that the out-of-body self can be projected from the body. The OBE has a biological function when it happens during life-threatening situations because when you think you are out of the body, [the body can then heal itself]. But the surviving self, the continuing self, the psychic self is not the out-of-body self. (Roll, 1995, pp. 118–119)

The subjects with whom I spoke had similar experiences to those of the subjects described in the parapsychology literature. The subjects showed remarkable lack of interest in activities that under normal circumstances would be of prime concern. The man, for example, who watched the staff try to revive him after he passed out during the stress test showed little concern for the survival of his body. Heather, the woman in labor, had to think about whether in her OBE state she was still pregnant. She also showed little or no interest in the labor process and her yet-to-be-born son. These were major concerns in normal life. The focus during OBEs often turns to things that are out of place or unknown in the situation.

I checked the veridicality of Heather's observation while in labor. She told me that she had never seen the doctor who had been called in to consult, either before or after the delivery experience. She did not even know his name. As part of the study, I pulled her medical record to verify her experience and found the name of the consulting physician. I then asked an obstetrician who would have known both men to describe them. He described them exactly the way Heather did, except that the consulting physician was a little taller than Heather's regular doctor. In addition, he said the consulting doctor was not part of the group of physicians Heather's primary doctor belonged to. There was no way she would have seen him during her regular visits.

What is interesting and not usually mentioned in the parapsychology literature is the consistency with which subjects report their observations from a view above the subjects. Heather, for example, reported the top of the head of the consulting physician. It would have been difficult from that position to determine who was taller.

Detection Studies

Other parapsychologists attempted what are commonly called detection studies. Attempts were made to use instruments and animals to detect the part of the person that left the body. According to Rogo, quite a bit of experimentation was carried out during the early years of psychical research, especially in France, on the instrumental detection of the human "double." The standard protocol was for the experimenter to mesmerize the subject, exteriorize his or her double, direct it to another room, and see if it could be photographed, produce raps, or illuminate specially prepared screens (Rogo, 1984). Several attempts were made at instrumentally detecting Harrary's OBEs. Instruments were placed in the target area. While Harrary was not successful at consistently affecting the detection devices, some readings did occur when he was projecting to the room. Some limited success was achieved by having human detectors present. Several researchers positioned known psychics in the target areas. Systematic work with these psychics was unsuccessful even though there were occasional accurate detections.

Animal detections were more promising. One of Harrary's pet kittens was placed in the target area. Harrary attempted two OBEs and imagined two others. In the two actual OBEs the kitten markedly decreased its activity and vocalizing. It became calm in Harrary's presence during the OBE. The results were significant at the .01 level. The research supporting the theory that OBEs involve something separating from the body is inconclusive but not easily dismissed. There were too many positive results to say definitely that something does not leave the body during an OBE. However, the results are not strong and consistent enough to prove something does leave the body.

THE PSYCHOLOGICAL THEORIES

A number of studies were done to test the psychological stability of subjects who had reported out-of-body experiences. Some of the initial beliefs held that OBEs were hallucinations caused by psychopathological conditions. The results of the psychological studies indicate that people who have OBEs are not remarkably different in any way. These experiences are evenly distributed between men and women. Also, education, socioeconomic status, and religious orientation do not make a difference (Green, 1968: Palmer, 1979; Gabbard et al., 1982).

In 1983, a group of researchers studied the personalities of individuals who reported OBEs (Myers et al., 1983). They found them to be responsible, honest, curious, inquisitive, adventure-seeking, clever, intellectual, analytical, social, and low in conformity. Some OBEs take place because of stress or physiologically compromised states. Others take place during relaxation or for no apparent reasons. Others take place during abuse when the abused person dissociates from the situation. Some of these abused subjects dissociate through OBEs.

While most of the subjects in this study had rather normal lives, one subject did report a childhood history of physical abuse by her mother. When her mother would beat her, she would go out of her body and watch from above what was happening to her. She felt comfortable and not in any pain while out of her body. During her hospitalization, she had a near-death experience (which will be reported in the next chapter). She also had an OBE, separate from the NDE, during which time she watched the doctors and nurses put tubes into her neck.

Harvey Irwin is a leading Australian researcher who believes that childhood trauma may be one of the psychological origins of paranormal belief. Irwin (1985) found a positive correlation between a global measure of paranormal belief and the incidence of traumatic events in childhood. Irwin's model proposes that childhood traumas evoke in the person a need for a sense of control over life events, and that by enhancing the appeal of paranormal ideas it enables the person to do that. Depersonalization or dissociation is seen as a mechanism by which subjects cope with severe stress. Patients with multiple personalities represent the extreme use of dissociation that is considered pathological. About 95 percent of patients with multiple personalities have a history of abuse. However, dissociation occurs in psychologically healthy individuals as well, We all "tune out" at times when the activity in our environment is boring or monotonous. Boring lectures, monotonous rides are classic opportunities for normal individuals to mentally leave the world and go into their heads to think about other things. The question about the relationship between dissociation and OBEs, however, is still unanswered. One of Irwin's studies did show that subjects who had OBEs were better able to immerse themselves in experiences to the exclusion of the outside world (Irwin, 1985).

Irwin in a later study demonstrated that children of alcoholics were more likely to believe in witchcraft, superstition, and precognition than children of nonalcoholics. His belief is that these children's home lives made them generally more receptive to paranormal belief. What is not clear is whether paranormal experiences are disassociative experiences and thus are unreal except in the mind of the experiencer, or whether the ability to dissociate enhances one's ability to have paranormal experiences and reach another state of reality.

BIOPHYSIOLOGICAL THEORIES

The one strong biophysiological theory is that OBEs are due to abnormal activity in the temporal lobe. Wilder Penfield (1955) produced OBE-like images through electrical stimulation of loci in the temporal cortex.

COMMENT

At this time there is no definite answer to the question "Does something leave the body during an OBE?" While all points of view have evidence to support their claims, none offers irrefutable proof. What is known is that severe pain and being close to death can provide a condition conducive to these experiences. Also, individuals who have these experiences do not have psychopathological characteristics. In my study, since a psychiatric history was an exclusion criterion, that was not a factor.

11

NEAR-DEATH EXPERIENCES

Eight patients from the Hartford Hospital study and three from the pilot study reported having a near death experience (NDE). Their experiences are generally consistent with those described in the literature (Moody, 1975; Ring, 1980; Greyson and Bush, 1992). Some subjects had only a few of the components of the NDE and others had many.

NEAR-DEATH EXPERIENCES

The first subject, Brian, was a 74–year-old man admitted because of an acute myocardial infarction.

Brian

"I was walking and felt these pains. I said to myself, 'I'm having a heart attack.' I remember praying to Jesus to take the pain away. Then I felt this relaxation, this feeling of contentment and euphoria like nothing I've ever experienced before. There was no pain. It was wonderful. I remember I was in a dark area and all I could see was this bright light in a room. I can't talk time, there wasn't any. I had no fear of dying. Then I felt pain. I'm back in the hospital room."

"Do you remember anything else?"

"I came back fighting. 'Why do I have to be here?' I said.

"How did this affect you?"

"I have no fear of dying."

Another subject was 61–year-old Curtis.

Curtis

"What was the last thing you remember before you became unconscious?"

"I had a cardiac arrest. I was going through a tunnel, more or less, clouds and all, feet first. They must have revived me. I said, 'What the heck is going on?' They must have put the paddles on me and brought me to. I didn't see anybody, just the clouds. This happened twice. The second time it was even a shorter distance. I went through the tunnel again. That's all I remember."

"What was your reaction to this experience?"

"I didn't believe it at first. At first I didn't think it actually happened. I thought it was possibly a dream, but then I said, 'No, it couldn't have been a dream. It actually happened. I was there.'"

"What was the difference between the experience and your dreams?"

"When you have a dream at home you say, 'This is a silly dream.' You are somewhere in Nova Scotia or in a different world, but in fact you are actually here. In this experience I was being treated for a heart attack. I was here. It was like putting two and two together. I had a brother-in-law and he went all the way. He spoke to the boss and told him he wasn't ready to go. He's the kind of person who doesn't throw any bull. He says it as it is. This is what happens in these circumstances."

Stanley was a 56–year-old man admitted with an acute myocardial infarction. The admission note said he had had ventricular fibrillation with a prompt response to defibrillation.

Stanley

"I was rushed into the ambulance and had another heart attack. I passed out. I remember seeing a round light. It was shimmering. I remember a really serene feeling came over me like 'Oh, this isn't so bad. This is going to be nice.' Then it disappeared. I came to because they put the paddles on me. The EMT said my heart had stopped. I was just shaking like a bowl of jello.

"All I remember was a very serene feeling. It was like 'This wasn't so bad to go. It is going to be nice.' I felt no aches, no pains. This is going to be all right. All my backaches were gone. I was hesitant to tell anybody about it at first. Then I told the doctor. He said I wasn't the first one to have that experience. I thought they'd probably lock me up in the loony bin."

"What do you think about this experience?"

"Personally, I had always poohpoohed these ideas, to be honest with you. When these shows came on TV, I always shut them off. Now I know they really happen."

Carrie was a 25–year-old woman admitted because of a diabetic coma.

Carrie

"I can remember some kind of like meadow and stream flowing through it. I don't remember flowers or trees or anything like that. I do remember this stream with some kind of crossing. There was a point where if I went past this I was not coming back. I don't remember a voice but I do remember somehow being told I couldn't cross the stream. It wasn't time for me yet. I don't know if it was telepathy, but I thought something like 'I don't want to go back. Can I stay for a while?' They said, 'OK.' They let me stay there and just kind of wander around. It was peaceful. It was quiet. Not harsh or bright. It was a nice place to be, and I was very happy there. I suppose something in me knew I had to go back, that I was eventually going back."

"Can you back up a little? The first thing you remember during this experience was the meadow and the river?"

"Yes, I just remember all of a sudden just being there."

"How did you feel when you were there?"

"I felt at peace. It was quiet, which was not common in my life at that time. There was a lot of love surrounding me. Everything was fine and everything was going to be fine. Even though my life was hell, someone was there watching me and it was OK, someone whom I understood to be God."

"Now, you said before you thought it was a they?"

"It felt like more than one being. Somebody was watching out for me, and it wasn't just one person."

"Was there some reason you wanted to stay?"

"There was no pain there. That was nice, peaceful. I told a nurse about it when I got back. She told me it was probably a dream. I got the impression if I pushed it, they might try to get me into the psychiatric ward. I was pretty sure that something important had happened. If it was going to get that kind of reception I wasn't going to say anything. It seemed safer not to say anything."

"Did it have any kind of effect on you?"

"It made quite a bit of difference. I knew I needed to go back to church. I needed to be responsible for me. I have since done a lot of charity work. Finding clothes for people who need them and giving them my mittens and stuff like that. Giving money to people. I just got married in June, and I'm not ready to go now. For once I am happy, but if I were to go I would be OK. No matter what some people say, there is a God and a Jesus and no one can take that away from me. I have seen them. I have been with them, and so I know that there is a nice place. I know they know me and accept me."

Eloise was 54–year-old woman in an ICU because of a subarachnoid hemorrhage. She had had a cardiac arrest in the ICU.

Eloise

"I was up toward the ceiling. I watched the doctors and nurses around my bed, checking the equipment, putting paddles on my chest."

"How did you feel when you saw your body on the bed?"

"Do you really want to know? All I could think of was to say to myself, 'Honey, do you need to lose weight."

"What did you look like up on the ceiling?"

"I honestly don't remember. I just felt like I always did. Like it was me up there. My body didn't really matter. I remember feeling wonderful, totally at peace. I saw this light and felt totally loved. Then I was back in my body. I tried to go back and have the experience again. I heard the male nurse yell, and I hated him for resuscitating me again. I wanted to go back."

Louis was a 60–year-old man who had his experience while undergoing open heart surgery.

Louis

"I was prepped for surgery. The doctor was looking at me and he says, 'You are going to feel a little pinch.' I felt the pinch and I'm waiting for him to tell me something more. I realize I'm no longer there. He didn't have to tell me, I could see him. I'm up at the ceiling looking down at him and the two doctors and a nurse assistant. I guess an anesthesiologist. I could look through those I didn't choose to see what they were doing. I could look through them and see the doctor's boots."

"You could see through the people?"

"I saw them and I looked at them, but then my vision penetrated through the corner of the stretcher. I told the doctor he wore glasses. I never knew he wore glasses. Anyhow, I became very uninterested in what they were doing."

"What were your reactions to being out of your body and seeing your body on the operating room table?"

"Kind of a who-cares attitude. I assumed the real me was up here. What I was looking at was something I used to travel in—like a

Stop and Shop bag or something similar. It just wasn't me because the real me was up watching. I didn't feel any compassion. I had no feeling for what was there. I was at first curious as to what they were doing.

"After making the decision that all of this was of no interest to me, I decided I should do something else. Upon making that decision to leave, immediately I was engulfed in total pitch black. I called it smoke that wouldn't leave. I was scared—it was totally foreign to me. It was something I had no knowledge of. Everything was black, and an entity came out of the blackness toward me. He looked like what we call the grim reaper. He was a skeleton with moving robes. I had never since seen a Halloween costume that spooky—a hand kept coming from the darkness like this. He was motioning for me to come toward him.

"Through telepathy he indicated to me that I should be heading toward the light. Now I had no idea what he meant by the light. I had heard of the tunnel and this kind of stuff but I never believed in that. I was supposed to go toward the light, and this guy is apparently going to show me. He swirled his finger and swirled a light area like a tunnel. It was a white area. He said to go in there, and I said no. That is not what I'm supposed to do. I think anyone with an IQ of a turnip would have known that was not a light. He just made a hole there.

"I refused to go, and all the darkness left. He left. I was in a domed lit area. Upon losing this darkness, I felt very peaceful. I was no longer afraid. I don't know how long I had been staying there. I felt great. This is not bad, but there must be something I am supposed to do. I was thinking I had to make some kind of journey.

"I looked upward and everything seemed to be brighter. I thought myself into an ascent. It wasn't swift, because I was unsure of where I was headed. I continued for miles, but it didn't take long. In front of me was a brown ceramic wall. Immediately upon hitting that barrier, I started to feel a love, a joy, a real euphoric feeling that I had never had. I felt loved. I felt as if I were really loved for the first time. When I turned my head I saw three figures—one was my deceased brother-in-law. I didn't know the other two guys."

"What did your brother-in-law look like?"

"Exactly as I knew him in his healthier days. He died of a heart problem. He looked pretty healthy."

"Did they have on clothes?"

"I couldn't see anything but heads. Faces—that was all I saw right there. I already learned you don't contact them through yelling. You communicate with them through your mind. I got excited about seeing him. He was my first point of reference. I started to yell his name. He just drifted away. I realized then that I was dead because he was dead. I still felt fine. I am dead, but this is grand. I was being bathed in this light all the time. Then I took an inventory of what I brought with me. This was bizarre. I had my head, my right arm, and my left leg. That's all I took with me, but I felt total. I felt connected but there was space in between my arm and my head.

"I don't know why but I had a need to get to the wall. On the other side was the most beautiful geography. Very rich brown, yellows. Everything was very rich looking. In the middle was this beautiful cauldron of light. All around it everything was very rich.

"Then my senses changed and I could hear every color. They gave off vibrations. I could hear and I could see peace and love. I could see an energy. From this bubbling energy a kind of brown wavy motion comes right up. It kept coming. It turned out to be my mother who died when I was seven years old. She was cloaked in brown—her favorite color, I later found out from my aunts. My first thought was, 'Are you my mother?' She retorted back telepathically, 'You are my son.' That was the answer. She started giving me knowledge. She gave me formulas. She gave me the cure for all of the nation's catastrophic ills. I accepted everything. How many things she told me I just can't remember because of restriction when you get back down here. Then she got a concerned look. She went from a warm, peaceful, smile to a look of concern. She started to float. I was concerned myself. 'Gee, my mom is leaving,' but I still felt loved. I looked at where she was going—she went to the operating room. There I am down there. The doctor is down there flapping his arms. He gestured and then began moving something out of the way. My mother grabbed his hands and she moved him and she came right back up to me.

I said, 'What was all of that?' She said, 'He was having a problem.' Oh, okay I accepted that. My brother-in-law comes back and starts telling me you have to go back and do some of the things your mother told you to do. 'No,' I said, 'I'm not going back. I'm having quality time with my mother. I'd just as soon stay here.' My mother gave me an acknowledgment that 'Yes, you have to leave.' In that instant a little boy seven or eight popped up right alongside me. Very gaunt looking, sparse hair, very tired. He was very puzzled. There was no one to help him, so I tried to reach him and hug him. I explained to him that he was dead but everything was okay. My mother gave me his name and said he was just on a visit but would be back in a couple of years. After this happened I went to visit the parents. I didn't say anything about the experience. The kids were fine. Subsequent to that the boy was taken to the hospital with a brain tumor.

"I remember being scared about coming back. My brother-in-law said to go another way. I thought myself into the operating room. Lo and behold, there I am. I am wide open. I've got something across my chest, something like a brace with clamps holding me apart. I knew I had to get back into my body. I decided to go in through the top of my head. I remember it feeling not tight. I settled down again and then total blackness."

"How has this experience affected you?"

"I have never been a bad person. I always liked people, but I never felt so badly for them. This compassion started taking over. I can't stand watching TV and seeing those kids that are starving. Coming home from the hospital there were a couple of kids out there and it was cold. It was so cold. I had a coat and I was so warm. I almost told my wife's uncle, 'Why don't you stop the car? I will let them have my coat.' I just felt that way. They probably would have run away. I felt like, 'I'm so warm why can't I give them my coat?'"

Fear of Death

Patients who have a near-death experience typically report no fear of death once they have recovered. However, I recently interviewed a patient, Bernie, who was terminally ill with cancer and had had a near-death experience eight years before our conversation. He had had a severe bleeding episode from an open vein in his nose, literally soaking several towels. He was admitted to the hospital and during the night went out of his body. He went through a tunnel that included white and pinkish-purple, puffy clouds that he described as "just beautiful." He started walking through the tunnel and saw a figure at the end of the tunnel that he believed was Jesus. The whole tunnel was "full of love," he said. The figure said he had to go back, it wasn't his time. Bernie said, "But I don't want to go back, I want to stay here."

I asked him how he felt about dying now that he had cancer and was in a hospice program. He said that while he hated leaving his family, he wasn't afraid to die. In fact, he looked forward to the experience. "I can't wait," he said.

NEGATIVE NEAR-DEATH EXPERIENCES

One of the patients interviewed had both a negative and a positive experience. Tim was 28 at the time of his accident.

Tim

"I was over at a friend's house having a good time. We were low on beer, so I went to get some. I remember my buddy's wife asking me not to go. I had been drinking a lot. I got on my motorcycle and wiped out a few miles down the road. I had this sensation of going down there into a hole. There was fire down there and figures. My father who had died was there. He told me it wasn't my time. Then he and I went up through a tunnel toward a light. I felt totally transformed. My father told me I had to go back. The next thing I remember I was in the hospital."

"How did this experience affect you?"

"I stopped drinking. I go to church now. It totally turned my life around."

OBSTETRICAL NEAR-DEATH EXPERIENCES

While there are some references to NDEs occurring in obstetrical patients, these experiences are not well-documented. The following are descriptions of two patients who had characteristic NDEs while delivering their babies.

Sally's experience happened a number of years ago while she was in labor with her son Robert. Sally had been given an epidural for anesthesia, which resulted in her blood pressure becoming severely low. Sally said she felt herself become distant from the events surrounding her. She felt a total feeling of peace, contentment, and joy. She lost all concern for what was happening to her body and, to her later chagrin, her unborn child. "It felt wonderful," she said.

Hillary was given medication for pain that lowered her blood pressure. She realized her unborn child was in distress.

Hillary

"I heard them talking about the baby's heart rate being low. The next thing I knew I was above everyone. I watched them scurrying frantically, checking my blood pressure, giving me oxygen.

I soon noticed a dark area and started walking toward it. I saw my mother who had recently died and was so happy to see her. She called me to her. As I started walking away, I looked back at my husband. I knew he would feel bad about me not being with him but I thought he would get over it. I assumed the baby had died. I started walking toward my mother again. I felt wonderful, totally at peace. Then I remembered my son Tod, who was four at the time. I knew I couldn't leave him. I had to go back to take care of him. The next thing I remember was being back in my body, feeling the labor pains. Soon my daughter was born. She was fine."

EXPLANATIONS

Near-death experiences have been described as long ago as the sixth century. Pope Gregory the Great in the sixth century wrote *Dialogues*, a collection of wonder tales that included reports of returns from death. While the tales included more accounts of hell than heaven—thus reinforcing the need to conform to church teachings—there were several elements of the modern NDE in these stories.

According to another early source, *The Book of the Dead*, during the dynastic period the Egyptians expected to enter the Judgment Hall of Osiris after death. They believed there they would begin an everlasting life. *The Book of the Dead*, which contains material gathered from every part of Egypt and the Sudan, revealed beliefs in the resurrection of a spiritual body, recognition of relatives and friends after death, and the continued existence of the heart-soul.

The ecclesiastical writings of the early Christians also included many accounts of communication with the dead and other paranormal events. In all these writings, death is regarded as transition or transformation and not as the final annihilation of the individual.

Since most of these sources were religious in nature, they were not seriously considered by members of the scientific community. In the late nineteenth century, the Canadian physician Sir William Osler was one of the first to carry out a medical investigation of this phenomenon. In a study of some 500 deaths, he concluded that only about 20 percent of the dying suffered emotional or physical pain. Albert Heim, the nineteenth-century Swiss geologist, was another investigator from the Cartesian-Newtonian materialistic view, which was the dominant theory at the time. After a near-fatal fall in the Alps, during which he had a mystical experience, he became interested in the subjective experiences associated with life-threatening situations. Over a period of several decades he collected observations and accounts from many survivors of serious accidents: soldiers wounded in battles, masons and roofers who had fallen from heights, and other accident victims, most importantly Alpine climbers who survived near-fatal falls. He first presented his findings in a paper read to a meeting of the Swiss Alpine Club in 1892. The experiences of the subjects he interviewed were similar in 95 percent of the cases. He reported the following characteristics of these experiences.

1. Mental activity first became enhanced and accelerated
2. Perception of events and anticipation of the outcome were unusually clear
3. Time became greatly expanded, individuals acted with lightning speed and accurate reality testing
4. Life review
5. Transcendental peace
6. Visions of supernatural beauty and the sound of celestial music

According to Hein, sudden confrontations with death were much more horrible and cruel for the observers than for the victims.

The contemporary interest in NDEs is credited to Raymond Moody, a psychiatrist and philosopher. His book *Life after Life*, published in 1975, contained anecdotal descriptions of 150 near-death experiences. Soon to follow in 1980 was Kenneth Ring's book *Life at Death: A Scientific Investigation of the Near-Death Experience*. Moody and Ring describe near-death experiences in similar ways. Typically patients feel euphoric, experiencing total lack of pain, anxiety, or stress. They describe themselves as feeling at peace and often characterize the event as their most wonderful experience.

If they go farther into the near-death experience, they often experience out-of-body events, telepathic communication, passage through a tunnel-like structure, encountering a light or a barrier, and a decision or charge to return to the "real world." Often, they arrive at this decision by interacting with dead friends or relatives whom they see during the near-death experience. Subjects who go deep into the experience report being given knowledge. Often that information is forgotten upon return but may be remembered when a situation presents itself. After the near-death experience, the experiencers report marked changes in their lives. They lose their fear of death and have a renewed sense of purpose. That purpose is directed toward helping others and a significant lack of interest in material goods.

Cross-cultural research shows that near-death experience is essentially the same whether it happens in India, Australia, or the

United States. Furthermore, demographics such as age, sex, race, social class, education level, and occupation have no effect on the incidence of NDE.

Not all experiences, however, were pleasant. Greyson and Bush (1992) reported on their study of fifty negative near-death experiences. These experiences often included hellish figures and painful and frightening visions. These researchers conclude that between 10 and 30 percent of all individuals who come close to death will have a near-death experience. Somewhere between 2 and 6 percent will be negative ones.

The explanations for NDEs include assessments that they are extrasensory experiences, psychologically induced, or biophysiological. The scientists who believe that NDEs are extrasensory experiences describe them as anomalies that our current paradigm of normal science cannot explain. William Serdahly, for example, believes that the paradigm of today's normal science needs to shift to accommodate the data from near-death studies. Since the publication of Moody's book, the number of anomalies has continued to mount. Several researchers have described not only the types of experiences that the subjects have but also the veridical perceptions during these experiences. One of the puzzles has been finding an explanation of how subjects can see what they report seeing while unconscious.

VERIDICAL PERCEPTIONS

Similar to the studies of OBEs not associated with NDEs, a trend in the research on NDEs has been that of the veridical perception of subjects. One of the best known studies was done by Michael Sabom (1982). Dr. Sabom, an Atlanta cardiologist, was initially very skeptical about NDEs. When he started talking to his patients, he was surprised at the number who reported them. In his research, Sabom compared the knowledge of resuscitation of 32 people who claimed to have observed their resuscitation while out of their body with 25 patients in a comparison group who had undergone resuscitation but had not had out-of-body experiences. None of the 32

subjects made major mistakes in describing the resuscitation procedure. In fact, they made some surprising observations. However,
23 of the 25 subjects in the comparison groups made major errors.

Following Sabom's study were reports of several cases involving corroboration of what was seen by subjects while out of their
bodies. Perhaps the most famous case of this kind is that of Maria,
originally reported by her critical care social worker, Kimberly
Clark (1984). Maria, a migrant worker, had a severe heart attack.
After a few days in the hospital, she developed more cardiac
problems and had a cardiac arrest associated with an unusual OBE.
At one point during this experience, she believed herself to be
outside the hospital, where she says she spotted a tennis shoe on
the ledge of the building. Maria not only indicated the whereabouts
of this oddly situated object, but she also described the little toe as
worn and one shoelace tucked underneath. These observations were
not possible from inside the room. Clark went to the location that
Maria had described and found the shoe precisely where Maria had
described it. Interestingly, Clark, from her point of view at the
window, could not see all the details Maria described. For example,
the worn small toe faced away from the window. Clark's conclusion
was that Maria could only have had such a perspective if she had
been floating right outside and at very close range to the tennis shoe
(Clark, 1984).

Ken Ring and I reported three cases that were similar to the one
described by Clark. In one case, a patient told a nurse that during
her resuscitation she had floated up over her body. She found herself
above the roof of the hospital, where she saw a red object that turned
out to be a shoe. The nurse told the woman's account to a skeptical
resident, who got the janitor to open the door to the roof. He came
back to the unit holding a red shoe. In the second case, a nurse from
the surgical intensive care unit was involved in the resuscitation of
a patient. The nurse, just back from vacation, was wearing a pair
of plaid shoelaces she had just purchased. The next day when she
went in to see the patient, he recognized her as the nurse with the
plaid shoelaces. A similar experience occurred to a respiratory
therapist. She was helping to resuscitate a man in his sixties in the

emergency room. He was being repeatedly shocked with no response, although he eventually recovered. When she saw him a few days later, he commented on how he liked her better in the yellow smock she had been wearing the day of his resuscitation (Ring and Lawrence, 1993). (This article is presented in total in the appendix.)

Ken Ring has recently completed a study of the NDE experiences of subjects who are blind, reported in more detail in Chapter 15. They, too, reported seeing. While several researchers believe these experiences cannot be explained by our current understanding of normal science, others believe the explanations are there. Paul Kurtz asserted that near-death experiences can be best explained by ordinary science, with the explanation residing in well-known phenomena such as hypnagogic or hypnopompic states (Kurtz, 1988). Saavedrea and Gomez (1989) described a neurobiological model for explaining near-death experiences based on temporal lobe dysfunction, hypoxia/ischemia, stress, and neuropeptides/neurotransmitter imbalance. The following is a description of the temporal pattern giving rise to NDEs.

1. A traumatic event, for example, cardiac arrest.

2. Appearance of brain stress.

3. Release of neuropeptides and/or neurotransmitter.

4. Decrease in oxygen tension in the brain, affecting mainly limbic structures.

5. Abnormal excitation of target tissues.

6. Epileptiform discharges in the hippocampus and amygdala.

7. Afterdischarge propogating through limbic connections toward more distant regions.

8. A recovery process, involving a rise in the rate of firing of inhibitory neuron, release of GABA, increase in O_2 tension, and energetic recovery.

The authors believe that in a given case the contribution of each of these factors could vary. Stress-induced release of B-endorphin is correlated with euphoria, analgesia, and long and lasting detachments. The entire model is based on the clinical similarities between temporal lobe seizures and NDEs.

Richard Blacher comments that while the authors emphasize that temporal lobe phenomena and near-death phenomena are very similar, it may be too narrow a focus to relate all near-death phenomena to the temporal lobe, since we are not dealing with demonstrable lesion of that lobe but rather with more general brain reactions (Blacher, 1972).

Rodin, a specialist in the treatment of seizures, made the following comment about the model. "In spite of having seen hundreds of patients with temporal lobe seizures during three decades of professional life, I have never come across that symptom [the components of the NDE] as part of a seizure. Furthermore, electrical stimulation of neocortical structures of the amygdala or hippocampus also failed to induce these symptoms. On the contrary, stimulation led to a sensation of fear and never of pleasure" (Rodin, 1989).

Susan Blackmore (1993) also thinks that normal science can explain the components of the NDE. She believes all the experiences can be accounted for by the dying brain. Anoxia accounts for the tunnel, and lights and endorphins induce the positive emotions. Studies have been done that show that endorphins are released at the time of death (Carr, 1981). However, the endorphin effect is usually short-lived, so the prolonged effect is not explained. Also, there is no explanation for why some patients who come close to death do not feel joy and peace.

Sherwin Nuland (1995) also believes the NDE can be explained by the evolution of normal science. "I believe the near-death experience is the result of a few million years of biological evolution and that it has a life preserving function for the species. My expectation is that it will one day be proved to be driven, if not specifically by endorphin, then by some similar biochemical mechanism. I would not be surprised if some of the other elements that have been thought to be possible causes do prove to play a role, such as the psychological defense mechanism called depersonalization, the hallucinatory effect of terror, seizures originating in the temporal lobes of the brains, and insufficient cerebral oxygenation" (p. 138).

PSYCHOLOGICAL THEORIES

Early on, some interpreted the NDE as a defense against the threat of death. it was proposed that persons faced with potentially inescapable danger and subsequent death produced a pleasurable fantasy which protected the individual from being paralyzed by emotional shock (Noyes, 1972).

Noyes and Kletti renamed this point of view in contemporary terms and conceived the NDE as a type of depersonalization (Noyes and Kletti, 1976).

In a study of characteristics of near-death experiencers, Ring found that they were more likely than non-near-death experiencers to have been abused as children. The difference was statistically significant. Since abused subjects often use dissociation as a defense mechanism, he believes dissociation is a factor in near-death experiences. However, unlike cases of multiple personalities, not even most near-death experiencers reported a history of abuse (Ring and Rosing, 1990).

Again there is some evidence to support the various explanations. None, however, is so conclusive that one explanation prevails over another.

12

NEAR-DEATH VISITS

A number of subjects who were close to death reported being visited by deceased friends and family members in their hospital rooms. These patients interpreted the visits as occurring for two reasons: to provide comfort or to take the patient with them to the afterlife.

NEAR-DEATH VISITS

Near-death visits can include a sense of presence, telepathic communication, or actual visualization of departed friends and relatives. Unlike near-death experiences, these apparitions occur in the experiencers' environment. Sixty-eight-year-old Trudy, who had had an acute respiratory distress, had such a visit.

Trudy

"I was in this bed [the hospital]. I don't think I ever saw my mother. I felt like she was calling me."

"Do you remember hearing her?"

"No, she did not say a thing. I felt her presence but didn't see her. I just felt her presence calling me. I said, 'Ma, please don't take me now. Let me enjoy my grandchildren. You enjoyed your grand-children.' My mother lived to be 98 years old. She did a lot of nice things with her grandchildren. She lived with me all the time. I was very close to her. She always felt like she needed me. I felt scared. I thought she was going to take me."

Another subject, Dan, also sensed the presence of his father. He said he could smell the chemicals with which his father had worked. He felt as if his father had come to comfort him.

Gretchen had a similar experience with her son, who had died a number of years before. She was 74 at the time and had been resuscitated in the emergency room.

Gretchen

"I was on the stretcher in the hospital. My son, Bill, was walking beside the stretcher holding my hand. He told me not to worry, that everything was going to be all right. He was with me, and I kept saying, 'What are you going to do about Christmas and the children?' He said, 'When you are feeling a little stronger we will talk about it. You tell me what else you want done and I will do it.' Just regular conversation."

"When you were talking to him at this point, what was your reaction?"

"I thought, well, the only thing I thought was you can always depend on Bill. Bill would be right here for me."

"Can you describe what you saw?"

"It was Bill, I could tell by his height and his build and his voice. It was very clear and very soft. He got very cross with me because I was crying, and he said, 'You know I can't stand to see you cry. Stop the crying.' It was like we were having a little conversation."

"Did you think it strange to have this conversation?"

"I didn't see anything unusual at that. Bill always said he would be there when I needed him. Evidently that was one of the times he thought I needed him."

Another woman, Esther, who was 47, came into the hospital because of an acute myocardial infarction. She had been defibrillated several times because of the severity of her dysrhythmias. She reported seeing her deceased father shortly after she was revived.

Esther

"I remember by father, who had passed away in 1984. He was standing there with a plaid shirt on. His hair was darker than it used to be. He was younger than he was when he passed away."

"Did you pick up any kind of communication or sense of what he was doing there?"

"No. He was just standing there."

"How did you feel? Did you have any reaction to seeing him?"

"That it was unusual that he was there. But he was somebody I knew when he died. I had a little more money than my mother or my father did. We had a signal if he wanted to talk he would call and ring my phone one or two times and hang up and I would call him. Two or three times that day there was a telephone ring that was interrupted. It was kind of like a static signal. Like it didn't ring full. It was a choppy ring. I remember I was vacuuming and I would go and put down the vacuum and answer the phone. There would be nobody there. I remember having visions of him lying on the floor with this gold sweater of his. He died later that day on the golf course wearing the gold sweater."

Another patient, 59–year-old Ronald, had gone into cardiac arrest at home and described this near-death visit to me.

Ronald

"I was with my son-in-law, and had gotten out of the chair I was sitting in and walked into the kitchen. I got light-headed, and that was the last thing I remember until waking up in the hospital—except for the experience."

"Which was . . .?"

"My brothers and my father—all deceased—were standing above me. I wasn't lying down—I was standing up—and they were above me, like in a cloud, and they were waving me to come on. They were talking, but I couldn't hear what they were saying. I couldn't make out the words. I could see them waving to me to come on, come, and I was saying no, no, I don't want to go."

"When you had the arrest and could see your father and brothers, were you out of your body?"

"No, I was still in my body . . . I felt that I was still myself, and I was still in my body, and I wasn't going to give it up. That was the resistance. At the time I knew I was resisting going with them. . . . I tell myself now that I didn't want to go because they were dead—that's my interpretation of it."

"How did they look?"

"They looked about the same as they did when they died. My father was quite elderly, and they were quite young. My mother was deceased, but she wasn't there, which is strange."

"Do you have any idea why?"

"I really don't know. She died a long time ago. Many years before them. So maybe that's it."

EXPLANATIONS

These apparitions now form a new category in the already extensive list of apparitions associated with death. No one previously has reported subjects seeing dead friends and relatives in their rooms who had not subsequently died. These experiences are similar, however, to death-bed visions and after-death apparitions, phenomena quite well described in the parapsychology literature.

The first charge from the Society for Psychical Research, which was started in 1882, was to Professor Henry Sidgwick to undertake the Census of Hallucinations Study. Professor Sidgwick and his associates surveyed 17,000 subjects and asked them the following question, "Have you ever, when believing yourself to be completely awake, had a vivid impression of seeing or being seen by a living being or inanimate object or of hearing a voice which impression as far as you could discover was not due to any external physical cause?" Ten percent of 1,684 individuals answered yes to that question. Of that number, 95 were collectively perceived, that is, more than one person saw the apparition. Out of this study came a description of four classes of apparitions: experimental cases, crisis cases, postmortem cases, and ghosts.

Also the investigators presented the general description of the apparitions.

Appear and disappear in locked rooms.

Vanish while being watched.

Sometimes become transparent and fade away.

Often seen and heard by some of those present but not by all.

Disappear into walls and closed doors and pass through physical objects.

People have put their hands through them and walked through them without encountering any resistance.

Leave no obvious physical traces behind them.

The following is a classical description by Sidgwick and his colleagues of an apparition that would be today classified as an after-death experience. "A man came out of an upstairs room, in which he had been alone, onto the landing, noting the time as he did so. He saw the apparition of an old lady, dressed like his mother, come out of another room on the same floor and descend the stairs. As he watched the figure going down, his wife came up the stairs and passed so close to the descending figure that she appeared to him to brush against it. But she had neither seen nor felt it. At precisely the same time the percipient's mother, dressed in outdoor clothes as the figure had been, died in another town" (Sidgwick, 1984).

One of the other earlier types of apparition reported is called death-bed visions, so aptly described in two books: *Peak in Darien Experiences* (Cobbe, 1882) and *Death-Bed Visions* (Barrett, 1926). In both these books the authors describe incidents of the terminally ill who saw and often spoke to individuals who had previously died. Often the visions appeared just before the subjects' deaths and brought a feeling of comfort to the subjects. The visions often reduced the fear of dying and facilitated the process by reducing anxiety and resistance. Frances Cobbe, the author of *Peak in Darien Experiences*, describes the following death bed scene witnessed by a physician.

> I was watching one night beside a poor man dying of consumption; his case was hopeless but there was no appearance of the end being very near; he was in full possession of his senses, able to talk with a strong voice and not in the least drowsy. He had slept through the day and was so wakeful that I had been conversing with him on ordinary subjects to while away the long hours. Suddenly, while we were thus talking quietly together, he became silent, and fixed his eyes on one particular spot in the room, which was entirely vacant, even of furniture: at the same time a look of great delight changed the whole expression of his face, and after a moment of what seemed to be intense scrutiny of some object invisible to me, he said to me in a joyous tone, "There is Jim." Jim was a little son whom he had lost the year before, and whom I had known well, but the dying man had a son still living, named John, for whom we had sent, and I concluded it was of John he was speaking, and that he thought he heard him arriving: so I answered, "No. John has not been able to come."
>
> The man turned to me impatiently and said, "I do not mean John, I know he is not here, it is Jim, my little lame Jim: surely you remember him?"
>
> "Yes," I said, "I remember dear little Jim who died last year, quite well."
>
> "Don't you see him then? There he is," said the man, pointing to the vacant space on which his eyes were fixed: and when I did not answer, he repeated almost fretfully, "Don't you see him standing there?"
>
> I answered that I could not see him, though I felt perfectly convinced that something was visible to the sick man, which I could not perceive. When I gave him this answer he seemed quite amazed, and turned round to look at me with a glance almost of indignation. As his eyes met mine, I saw that a film seemed to pass over them, the light of intelligence died away, he gave a gentle sigh and expired. He did not live five minutes from the time he first said, "There is Jim," although there had been no sign of approaching death previous to that moment. (pp. 290–291)

The reports in Sir William Barrett's book on death-bed visions are similar. "An old man, named John George, lay dying. He and his wife, MaryAnn George, had had a great sorrow that same year in the death of their youngest son, Tom, a young man who had been killed on the railway line on which he worked. The dying man had been quiet some time as though sleeping, when he suddenly looked up, opened his eyes wide, and looking at the side of the bed opposite to where his wife was, exclaimed, 'Why, Mother, here is Tom, and he is all right, no marks on him. Oh, he looks fine.' Then after another silence, he said, 'And here is Nancy, too.' A pause, then, 'Mother, she is all right. She had been forgiven.' And very soon after he passed away, taking with him a sorrow which had long pressed upon the mother's heart, for Nancy had fallen into sin, and had died soon after the child was born, and as the poor mother thought, never having had time to repent."

Karlis Osis (1961), in a more contemporary study, surveyed doctors and nurses, asking them what percentage of patients they believed had had visions at the time of death. The respondents reported that about 10 percent of all patients reported these visions. When I have spoken to various groups of hospice nurses, they have indicated that number to be higher, somewhere between 50 and 75 percent. It may be that the recent social acceptance of matters like the near-death experience may improve the willingness to now talk about these types of occurrences.

Near-death visits are a variation of deathbed visions and after-death experience. In near-death visits, the subjects are not actively dying like those who experience death-bed visions. However, they have been close to death, unlike those who experience after-death experiences who are healthy but often grief stricken. According to research using the biomedical model, the feeling of a presence or the experience of postmortem apparitions has been thought to be due to changes in melatonin levels and/or a specific pattern of electrical activity within the deep mesiobasal (hippocampus and amygdala) structures and adjacent cortical regions of the left temporal lobe. M. A. Persinger (1993) analyzed the incidence of psi experiences through data presented in the *Fate Magazine* collection. He concluded through his analysis that most spontaneous psi experiences occur at night; 39 percent of the cases of telepathy, 37% of precognition cases, and 54 percent of postmortem apparitions. When he correlated these cases with the times melatonin is maximally elevated, there was a significant correlation between the time of the psi experiences and the melatonin elevation (.69 to .42).

Fate Magazine typically asks readers to write in and describe their experiences. While the editors are credible, they do not pretend that *Fate* is a scholarly journal. The data from the subjects about the incidence of psi phenomena were not scientifically obtained. Also, the correlations Persinger reported are moderate. Correlations only show relationships; they are never used to establish causality. At best, Persinger has presented an idea worth pursuing, but he does not prove that nocturnal melatonin levels are the precipitating source of experiences of postmortem apparitions, as he states.

Persinger participated in two other studies that indicated a correlation between the feeling of a presence and elevated temporal lobe function. Interestingly, these experiences did not occur at night during the hours of 12:00 A.M. and 6:00 A.M. as reported in the study discussed above (Persinger and Fisher, 1990; Persinger and Makarec, 1992).

In 1994, Lindal et al. did a study to determine the qualitative difference of visions and visual hallucinations. They analyzed the frequency and quality of visions in a general population of 862 subjects and 19 schizophrenic patients. Significant and qualitative differences were found in visions experienced by the members of the two groups. The general population most commonly experienced visions of people, whereas the schizophrenic patients were more likely to experience other phenomena. The authors conclude that these two experiences were qualitatively different and that visions were a different experience from hallucinations.

Parapsychologists have described two aspects to apparitions that are unexplainable and offer some evidence of the veridicality of apparitions. When two subjects see the same apparition, the parapsychologists compare each person's description for consistency. A number of death-bed visions included apparitions of persons who had died but were not known to the dying person as dead. Barrett described the case of a young woman who lay dying after childbirth. She reported seeing her father, who she knew had died. Shortly after that, she reported seeing her sister, who had died three weeks previously. She had not been told of her sister's death because of her serious illness.

This type of experience occurred with a patient at the hospital who had had a near-death visit from his mother and sister. His sister had died, but the patient's wife had insisted this be kept from the patient since he himself was so ill. When he asked about his sister, he was told she was fine. He kept insisting that he knew she was dead because he saw her with his mother and knew they were both deceased. A nurse also reported an afterdeath apparition that occurred to her and her mother, who were both driving in separate cars to meet each other. On the way, they passed the same street corner and both saw the nurse's grandmother on that corner. They both described her and what she was wearing in the same way.

For these cases, there is only limited evidence to support preliminary hypotheses. It seems clear that these visions are different from the hallucinations described in Chapter 8. However, a definitive explanation is still lacking.

13

THE GRIM REAPER

Three of the subjects I interviewed saw apparitions that they described as the grim reaper. Visions of the grim reaper were the only type of apparition seen that did not occur in normal life; all the other encounters described by the subjects had been or were currently present in everyday experiences. The subjects found the apparitions of the grim reaper to be frightening and very disconcerting.

The biggest surprise in conducting this research project was finding subjects who described their encounters with the grim reaper. The first subject was a middle-aged man, Ralph, who had had a strange experience and didn't know how to put it in a meaningful perspective.

Ralph had been admitted because he had had a heart attack. The last thing he remembered was having a doctor talk to him about a special medication. The next thing he remembered was feeling very cold—"below freezing," as he described it. "At the foot of my bed on the right side was a dark, gray, cloaked stranger. He had no face."

"How did you know it was a 'he'?"

"I don't know. I just knew. The other thing I knew was he didn't think I was bad enough or sick enough to go with him."

Ralph saw the figure as a hellish representation. He kept commenting on how cold he felt. He wasn't sure what it meant. Another patient reported an encounter with the grim reaper during a near-death experience. "I was the real Louis. There was nothing spiritual about me. Down there was the old thing I traveled in—the carrying case that used to tote me around. I was the real Louis, up here."

"Then what happened?"

"After making the decision that all of this was of no interest to me, I decided that I should do something else. I didn't know what else to do, but watching operations was not one of them. Upon making that decision, BAM. Immediately I was engulfed in total, pitch black—the total absence of any color. I was scared. It was totally foreign to me. And then this entity came out of the blackness toward me, looking like what we'd call the grim reaper."

"What did he look like?"

"Skeletal. Yellowish. And it had moving robes. Now, I could've been conditioned to see something like that, but I never saw a Halloween costume that spooky. And there was a hand coming from the darkness, motioning for me to come toward it—toward the entity."

"What was your reaction?"

"I was frightened. But I was also thinking, 'Well, he's the only thing I can identify here. The rest is total black.' So I thought that maybe I should pay attention to his directions, until I began to feel that he was trying to trick me into doing something other than what I'm supposed to do. And through telepathy, he indicated to me that I should be heading toward the light. Now, I had no idea what he meant by the light, other than maybe as a child I remember hearing about that stuff where you go through a tunnel and everything, but I never believed in any of that. I always thought it was all hooey until then. But he said I should be going toward the light, and I thought that he was making some sense."

"Can you describe him in a little more detail?"

"A skeleton. A skull . . . incessantly chattering. The teeth moving all the time. It was yellowish, with the typical black eyes. There was a black cloak, constantly moving. It was illuminated by its yellowishness. The hands were skeletal—just bones—and motioning for me to come toward it.

"Then he swirled his hand in the air," Louis said, as he made a circular motion with his own hand, "and made kind of a light area, like a tunnel. And he said, 'Go in there,' and I said no. That wasn't what I was supposed to do. I think anyone with the IQ of a turnip would have known that it wasn't a real light. He just made a hole there, and out of nowhere, he produced some yellow, acrid-looking stuff that he threw in the hole and swirled it around. And he said, 'You have a golden light. Go to it now.' But I refused.

"And when I refused, the darkness left, and I was in a domed, lit-up area, like an amphitheater. Everything just lightened up, and I wasn't scared anymore, just hanging in this area."

During talks that I have given to various groups, I have had three members of the audience report on similar experiences. A nurse said that one of her patients had seen the grim reaper. The patient had had a heart attack. He told her he saw this dark, hooded figure. In that patient's case, the Reaper had opened a door for the subject to enter. A student reported that his friend's father saw the reaper right before he died. The man was frightened and didn't know what seeing him meant. Another participant at a different lecture said that she herself had seen the reaper when she was a little girl. "I was 6 1/2 and very sick. My parents were very worried. I heard the doctor tell my mother that I could die. I was at a crisis in my illness. As I lay in this state, very weak and tired, I saw death at the foot of the bed. He was tall, skeletal, with a black cape over his head. He had big hollow spaces for eyes. He had a staff. He didn't move or talk. I was frightened but not terrified. I kept saying I didn't want to go. I was coughing very hard. A glob of stuff came out. The doctor said I was at the end of the crisis. I was going to make it. The image faded away. He faded very slowly. His head was first and the cape was the last thing to go."

As puzzling as these events are, another patient had an experience that makes these circumstances even more mystifying. This patient had a bleeding episode that precipitated a near-death experience. As the subject passed through the tunnel, he was overwhelmed with love and peace. At the end of the tunnel stood a figure with a bright light behind him. The figure was cloaked in a cape that was purple, almost black. The figure had no face. The subject said he knew it was Jesus. He felt his love. The figure told him he had to go back. In this case, the man interpreted the figure obviously very differently. In the last case, the environment was full of love and warmth. In the other situations, the subjects reported feeling coldness.

EXPLANATIONS

Only in a paranormal magazine called *Fate* did I find any reference to experiences with this mythical figure. As popular a mythical figure as the grim reaper is, the descriptions were very limited. Even an extensive search by the research librarian at the Parapsychology Foundation in New York turned up only these descriptions in *Fate* magazine.

In July, 1992, Mark Chorvinsky, the editor of *Fate*, published letters received from readers about their experiences with the grim reaper. One woman reported seeing, with a friend—when she and her friend were between eight and ten years old—a black-faced, hooded figure matching the description of the classic grim reaper. The entity glided up the road. The children watched it for several minutes until it disappeared. The entity had nothing but darkness inside the hood, according to the observers.

In another report a 50–year-old woman was awakened in the middle of the night by someone or something shaking her by the legs. She moved her legs but the tugging became stronger. "Sleepily, I opened my eyes," she said. "I became aware of a figure in a light-colored robe, its head covered in shadow, standing at the foot of my bed, leaning over while shaking my legs. My mind was cloudy with sleep. In the befuddled state I thought it was my mother in a bathrobe with a towel on her head. I called out, 'Ma, what is it? Are you all right?' Then the figure lifted its head. The figure had no face but was hooded." In a telepathic manner, the figure spoke to her. "I heard it inside my head and not with my ears, It said, 'Come with me—it's time to go!'" According to the article, all the woman then remembered was getting out of bed. She felt the figure touch her elbow . . . and had the impression that she and the reaper left through the window (Chorvinsky, 1992).

Another woman named Mrs. P. wrote in response to the first woman's letter. Early one evening, when she was between eight and ten, she went running up the stairs and saw, in the dim light, what she now recognizes as the grim reaper. "He was just standing there holding his scythe upright in his right hand. I remember turning back and sitting on the sofa gripped with fear. I never told anyone about this and I was afraid of the dark and other things for many years."

In May of 1993, Mr. Chorvinsky published more descriptions from his readers of encounters with the grim reaper. One reported an encounter with the reaper while dreaming. In that dream, a black figure, characteristic of the grim reaper, began a threatening descent. "By then I was real mad and raised my arm either to hit it or push it away. The strangest thing was that I could feel it. I touched it to push away. Halfway between sleep and waking, the reaper was actually hit with my hand and my hand did touch it like it was real."

Sometimes the reaper has been seen as a helpful figure. Mr. L. was stretched out on the sofa one evening when he had the sensation that someone was watching him. "I slowly glanced to my right and there he was standing at my side, holding his scythe upright. His face was a gleaming white skull. He was just looking at me. Then fear came over me. . . . , I said aloud, 'Who sent you to me? Go back to where you came from.' With that command he glided slowly backward, watching me the whole time. He never took his eyes off me. He never turned his back to me. When he reached the front door he went right through it and was gone. For a while I just stayed there thinking of what had happened. Why did he come to me and I'm still alive? I jumped up and ran to our bathroom thinking he could have come for someone else and I was too late. I called out to my wife and shook her. She was out cold with an empty bottle of pills on the bed. She tried to take her life. I tried harder to wake her by walking her - slapping her. She was not responding. I called my sister who lives nearby. We drove her to the hospital. She was released a week later. We went on with our lives." When Mr. L had time to process this experience, this was what he concluded. "The encounter has left me with the feeling that the reaper is a special friend. He appeared to me and gave warning instead of taking someone."

The next description from a *Fate* reader has some remarkable similarities to a description given by a patient interviewed for the Hartford Hospital study. Ms. V's father was in a hospital. He had been sick with cancer for many months. While watching him sleep one night, she remembers that he woke up and looked at her and asked for a drink of water. "I got up to get him the water. I was beside him when I heard him in a panic say to me, 'Please, help me—don't let him get me. Please keep him away from me!' I turned and looked around the room and saw no one. I said, 'Who, Dad? What are you talking about?' He said, 'Look over there, don't you see him?' I said, 'No, Dad, describe what you see.' He described to me a tall man, with a black robe and a hood—with his arms outstretched. He couldn't see a face or eyes but he knew it was a man."

Her brother told her of a similar experience with their father about a month later. Their father had told him of a hooded, black-robed figure. "My dad was very afraid. But my brother said he didn't see anything and he just felt cold."

As popular a mythical figure as the grim reaper is, there is little written about him. Surprisingly there is no book entitled "The Grim Reaper" describing its origin or other characteristics. Briefly, we know that the figure originally was a skeletal figure used primarily in the Middle Ages to portray death in paintings. Somewhere later in history, the figure acquired a cloak and then a scythe. It is interesting that Christ was portrayed as being cloaked and with a staff. Is it possible that the portrayal of the two figures—the skeletal death representation and the Christ figure—blended in history? This type of encounter is another area for which there is no known explanation.

14

PRONOUNCED DEAD BUT STILL ALIVE

During the data collection phase of this project, one patient caught the attention of many of the hospital staff. The woman had been pronounced dead after a code and "returned to life." I went to see her and found that she was willing to talk about it.

Louise was a 56–year-old woman who had come to the emergency room because of a severe asthma attack. She progressed to severe respiratory distress and ultimately to an electromechanical dissociation (EMD) arrest. A code was announced, and for over twenty minutes the code team attempted to resuscitate her. While there was some electrical activity on the monitor, the heart was not responding because of the disconnection. For more than twenty minutes she had no pulse and no blood pressure. Her breathing was supported by a ventilator. All the monitoring equipment indicated that Louise was not responding to any of the resuscitation attempts, so the code was stopped and all the equipment was shut off. The doctor called the family and began filling out the death certificate. Ten minutes later, as the nurse prepared Louise to be seen by the family, she started breathing on her own. In a flurry of excitement, the equipment was reapplied, and efforts to support her life continued.

Louise agreed to be interviewed. She was alert and oriented, with no obvious side effects from oxygen deprivation. Louise described what had happened to her during the time she had "died."

"The last thing I remember is that people were calling my name—but they were very far away."

"Who were the people?" I asked her.

"I don't know. Maybe it was the nurse. It was dark. I was walking to this place, but I wasn't sure where I was. And then I saw a coffin."

"A coffin?"

"I knew the coffin was mine. I didn't know where the room was, but I knew it was my coffin. And I also knew that it wasn't my time to go."

"How did you know that?"

"There were two people in the room, a man and a woman. Eric was a friend of my son Steve. He died three or four years ago of AIDS. Grace was my friend. She died this past year. There was a light around both of them. Eric did most of the talking, but they both told me that I was going to be fine—that it wasn't my time yet. They said I had to go back."

"How do you feel about this experience?"

"Okay."

"Okay?"

"Well, this happened to me before—seeing people who have died, years ago when Steve was only a boy of about nine or ten. I had another bad attack. Almost died that time, too. But that time, I kind of went out of my body, you know. I could see myself lying there. I saw a real bright light. Marian was there."

"Another friend of yours?"

"Yes. She had died, too. Before me. Said that it wasn't time—that I had to go back."

"Just like this time?"

"Sort of. That time I knew why I had to come back, to take care of my three kids. This time, I don't know what I'm supposed to do."

"What do you mean?"

"I don't know what my purpose is this time—why I was supposed to come back."

"How did you feel about coming back?"

"It was such a beautiful experience. The most beautiful experience ever. I didn't want to leave. I'm not afraid to die. I haven't been for a long time, since the first time I nearly died."

CLINICAL DEATH VERSUS BIOLOGICAL DEATH

Strange as it may seem, it actually is not a rare occurrence for someone to be pronounced dead and then come back to life. It has been reported that the fourteenth century Italian poet Peliah had been laid out in death. He would have been buried in four more hours but for a sudden change of temperature which caused him to sit up and complain of the draught. He lived another thirty years to write some of his best work.

In eighth-century England the monk Bede, in his *History of the English Church and People*, told the story of a man called Cunningham who had died in the early hours of the night. At daybreak, he returned to life and suddenly sat up, to the great consternation of those weeping around the body, who ran away. Cunningham described leaving his body to find himself in heavenly realms, accompanied by "a handsome man in a shining robe," and was not at all happy to be told he had to go back to the land of the living. "I was most reluctant to return to my body, for I was entranced by the pleasantness and beauty of the place. But I did not dare to question my guide and meanwhile I suddenly found myself alive amongst men once more" (Wilson, 1987, p. 111).

In 1949, former Army captain Oddment Wilbourne, an Englishman, "died" of pleurisy in Crumpsall Hospital, Manchester. After his doctor had declared him dead, a nurse made his body ready for the morgue. Unknown to her, Wilbourne was watching from a vantage-point out of his body.

"I can still picture the scene. I saw myself lying on the bed. I saw a young nurse. She was preparing me for the mortuary. I remember thinking at the time how young she was to have to do such a thing as getting me ready and even shaving me. I actually saw it taking place. I was detached from it, it was as if I were there watching and I was the third party. I felt no emotion, just nothing, like looking at a picture. I was clinically dead about two hours and I woke up at the mortuary of Crumpsall Hospital, and it was the mortuary attendant who nearly had a heart attack! I know it wasn't a dream" (Wilson, 1987, p. 114).

While it is not inconceivable that limited assessment instruments in earlier times could have led to confusion about the state of the patient, these occurrences still happen in our present times with sophisticated assessment equipment. In June of 1993 there was a front-page news story in New York City. A 40–year-old woman, a school teacher from Brooklyn, who had collapsed in her apartment, was declared dead by the emergency medical technician. Left as dead for several hours, she was later found to be alive. On June 21, 1993, Forrest Sawyer on ABC's "Day One" interviewed the Brady family, who had experienced yet another death pronouncement. In January 1992, Emma Brady was pronounced dead in a Florida hospital. Already in a body bag, she was ready to be taken to the morgue. Her head was sticking out—she was gasping for air. Her husband went to the hallway, looking for a nurse and asking, "Could you tell me, is that what a dead person is supposed to look like?" The nurse asked him if he would like a cup of coffee. Eventually, two nurses came in and checked the patient's blood pressure. They ushered the family out to the waiting room and later came back to tell them Mrs. Brady was indeed alive. The woman later reported that she knew she was being resuscitated, she knew they were beating on her chest and she knew that they were wrapping her up like a baby.

Carla Woods was declared dead by ambulance workers and the coroner's office. She also remembered the event. "I could hear people talking and moving around, and I got a really bad feeling. I tried to talk, and I couldn't talk. Nobody could hear me. I remember being wheeled somewhere—I could hear the wheels." The wheels Carla had heard were on the cart taking her to the morgue, where someone put a block under her head to lift it up. It was then that they noticed some movement in her throat and she was rushed to the emergency room. She suffered no permanent physical damage. However, she was emotionally traumatized. "I have had nightmares for years about being in the total darkness, being buried alive, screaming, yelling, no one hearing me. I'd wake up clawing, just, oh, terrible nightmares. I was afraid to sleep. I was afraid I wouldn't be able to wake up."

A Connecticut newspaper printed a story describing a man who had "died" in an area hotel room. The paramedics came and pronounced him dead, a pronouncement which was reaffirmed by the coroner. The patient subsequently began to breathe on his own. A student in our nursing program happened to work in the hospital to which he was brought. I helped her with a paper describing the patient's experiences. During the time the paramedics and the coroner were pronouncing him, he also had a classic near-death experience in which he was told it wasn't his time to die.

Currently, there is much discussion about clinical death versus biological death. The explanation for these cases is the inability in the clinical setting to predict that biological death has taken place. It is believed that while clinically patients can appear to be dead, biologically they are still alive. The point still can be made, however, that in most cases the detection methods we normally use in the hospital are generally adequate to detect death. While mispronouncements happen, they are, in fact, rare. The question still remains: what is it about these patients that makes them look clinically dead and yet has them revive spontaneously when all resuscitation efforts have failed?

In Louise's case, we have documentation of cardiac output, blood gas readings, and so forth, all of which indicated she was not responding to any treatment. There are no clear-cut answers to her spontaneous recovery.

15

CONCLUSIONS, CURRENT RESEARCH, AND CLINICAL IMPLICATIONS

The core of this book is the patients' descriptions of their experiences while unconscious. These descriptions portray better than any other method what the patients felt, thought, and perceived. The related research, underlying assumptions, paradigms, and theories have been included to describe what we currently know or don't understand about these experiences and to guide further research and interventions for these patients. The following are my general conclusions that have served to guide me when I have been in consultation with patients and families.

GENERAL STATEMENTS ABOUT THE NATURE OF THE EXPERIENCES

Being physiologically compromised is a necessary but not sufficient condition to cause the various experiences described by patients. All the patients were physiologically compromised. However, the same physiological condition did not result in the same response. For example, some patients in a cardiac arrest situation reported nothing; others said that they could hear when it was presumed that they could not. Some had internal dialogue; some went out of their bodies. There were patients who had near-death experiences or a near-death visit. The variety of experiences are inconsistent with our general knowledge of the body and how it functions. We in the health care field function on the consistency principle: the body will respond the same way given the same physiological conditions. We make the assumption in our journal articles, textbooks, and daily practices that in a cardiac arrest situation similar body responses are going to happen to patients, that is, the blood gas values will change in a predictable fashion. It seems that factors beyond the physiological processes determine the type of experiences a patient will have when unconscious.

Hearing is not the last sense to go, consciousness is. From their descriptions, the subjects reported being able to have internal dialogue even when they could hear no external information. When their bodies were not functioning and were being resuscitated, their consciousness was still functioning. One man was able to dream during a cardiac arrest. Even though the subjects were able to perceive, see, and emotionally respond during their out-of-body and near-death experiences, their ability to hear was gone. They reported receiving messages telepathically, not hearing them. Hearing, as we understand it, departs before the other senses and consciousness do.

Deteriorating biomedical processes are necessary but not sufficient conditions to cause death at some times during life. Death is not controlled solely by biomedical processes during some times of life. Positive energy from those near the dying person, the sense of purpose, and possibly a higher power are all factors that contribute to the life or death of an individual.

Hallucinations, illusions, and delusions differ from extrasensory experiences. When having hallucinations, illusions, and delusions, the subjects did not describe real phenomena. Nor were there consistent patterns to their experiences. In the out-of-body and near-death experiences, the subjects described what was happening in their environment. These descriptions—for example, the red shoes on the roof of the hospital—correlated with what was actually happening. There was also a consistent pattern to all these experiences. With remarkable consistency, patients who reported NDEs described being out of their bodies, going through a tunnel, and seeing dead friends or relatives. These patterns do not occur with hallucinations and illusions.

Patients, when unconscious, are able to feel the emotional energy of the people around them. Patients seem more sensitive to energy transfer during the unconscious state. First of all, patients reported being able to distinguish between negative, positive, and impoverished energy emanating from those around them. They reported being energized by positive, caring emotions that resulted in their increasing desire to get well. They reported being drained by negative and impoverished energy that often led to a lessening of consciousness or increased agitation.

The diminution of the functioning of the conscious mind through highly compromised physiological states or highly emotional states with a moderate compromised physiological state increases the opportunities for extrasensory experiences to occur. What blocks us from having extrasensory experiences is the conscious mind, which is controlled by the functioning of our physical body systems. When the physical body system is compromised through severe physiological conditions like a cardiac arrest, or a combination of a highly emotional state and moderately compromised physiological state, such as labor and delivery, when patients might have a drop in blood pressure, the conscious mind is replaced by another system that permits extrasensory experiences to happen. To a lesser degree, subjects who meditate or are more internally focused are able to block out external stimuli and concentrate on gaining access to these extrasensory experiences. Most of the subjects in this study were unsophisticated in the art of meditation or extrasensory experiences. Most were shocked by these experiences and could not understand what was happening to them. I believe that when the conscious mind became curtailed, these experiences just naturally happened.

*Some perceptual changes during the extrasensory experiences
are consistent for all subjects.* During extrasensory experiences, the
subjects typically reported receiving information telepathically.
The subjects who were not familiar with parapsychology did not
know to use the word telepathy. Their comments were more descriptive of the experience. It was not unusual for such a patient to
say he heard the conversation in his head. I think it is curious that
hearing changes during the extrasensory experiences. That implies
some body changes that interfere with our ability to pick up
auditory vibrations. Yet a few subjects reported hearing beautiful
music, the likes of which the subjects had never heard before.

*Apparitions of the grim reaper are the major anomaly of the
extrasensory experiences.* The grim reaper is a mythical figure,
symbolic and not real. All the other descriptions in the extrasensory
experiences were of real, or once real, people or events. I believe
any explanations of the other extrasensory experiences, whether
those explanations are biomedical, psychological, or parapsychological, would not also be able to explain the grim reaper.

RESEARCH IMPLICATIONS

This book has included the results of a research project on
unconscious patients along with related research studies. This
chapter includes research on aspects of unconsciousness that has
just been completed, is being conducted, or could be done. The
intent of this section is to describe approaches to further the
exploration of this type of research.

Veridical Perception Studies

In the past few years, some attempts have been made to test
the veridical perception of subjects who have had out-of-body
and/or near-death experiences that are naturally occurring. When
Michael Sabom, the Atlanta cardiologist (reported in Chapter 11),
compared the description of the resuscitation efforts of the patients who had been resuscitated but did not report experiencing

an NDE with those who reported experiencing an NDE during resuscitation, and showed the NDE group to be more accurate, he conducted one of the first veridical perception studies of hospitalized patients.

In the late 1980s, Janet Holden, Ed.D., posted cards with numbers and symbols high on the wall of a cardiac intensive care unit. The cards faced the ceiling so that no one could see them unless he was literally out of his body. Although it had been predicted that 10 percent of the patients in the unit would have an NDE, in a period of five months only one reported having such an experience. Holden stopped the study but hopes to reestablish it in another hospital.

Ken Ring, with an associate, Sharon Cooper, is in the process of completing a research study about blind near-death experiencers. He had three research questions: Do blind people have NDEs? Are they the same or different from the NDEs of sighted experiencers? Can they see during this experience? If they can see, can we corroborate what they saw? Ring and his associate were able to find 31 subjects to interview. Sixteen of these subjects had NDEs, four had an NDE and one or more OBEs, and eleven did not have an NDE but had one or more OBEs. Fourteen were blind from birth, twelve became blind later in life, and five were considered legally blind. At an Internation Association of Near-Death Studies (IANDS) conference in the summer of 1995, Ring reported on the subjects who described what they perceived to be sight. Because these experiences happened years before the research study was conducted, it was difficult to corroborate what each subject said he saw while he was out of his body. One man, for example, said he saw a necktie that his girlfriend had left at his house. He was able to describe the tie in great detail even though no one had had the opportunity to describe it to him. His girlfriend, unfortunately, only had a vague recollection of the event.

One of Ring's other subjects happens to be a personal acquaintance of mine and had a very detailed near-death experience. He was blind from birth and became very ill at the age of eight. He reported being out of his body and "seeing" people running to get help for him and then being outside "seeing" the lights and traffic in the streets. While he was further into the experience, he reported "seeing" very green grass and trees. One of the trees was a palm tree. When asked how he knew it was a palm tree, he replied he didn't know that was what it was at the time. Later, when he was about sixteen, he was in Florida and reported touching a palm tree and having someone describe it and name it. It was then that he could label the tree he saw during his NDE.

The issue of lack of validation of what is seen during these experiences brings up the problem of retrospective research studies. Unlike the parapsychologists who had their subjects induce out-of-body experiences, we obviously cannot recommend inducing near-death experiences. However, we know from previous research that a certain percentage of patients undergoing a type of cardiac study will have a near-death experience. That led me to do a prospective study at Hartford Hospital using subjects undergoing electrophysiology (EP) studies. In an EP study, a cardiologist induces the dysrhythmia that might seriously affect the patient during normal activities. The procedure involves the actual stimulation of the heart muscle by a catheter in the heart. The patient is tested with various medications to control the abnormal heart rhythm. From a previous study, we learned that 30 percent of all EP patients became unconscious during the procedure and needed to be defibrillated. Of that 30 percent, 9 percent reported having a near-death experience.

As a part of the prospective design, I gave a personality inventory and a Dissociative Experience Scale to patients before they went to have these EP studies. The purpose of administering these instruments was to see if personalities did change after an NDE, and to see if the tendency toward dissociation was a predicter of someone having an NDE or OBE. In addition, I placed an electronic sign high on a cabinet in the room, not visible to anyone standing on the floor. In order to read the sign a person needed to use a ladder or be out of his body. It contained a nonsense statement like, "The popsicles are in bloom," and I changed it randomly. It was nonsense so that no one could say he overheard a conversation about the words on the sign. All subjects who became unconscious during the EP studies were interviewed and asked to describe their experiences. We were hoping they had had an NDE and had read the sign.

The plan was then to administer the instruments six months later to patients who reported an NDE. It was hypothesized that personality score would change six months after the NDE. In the year the sign was in place, no one reported a full NDE while undergoing the EP study. Only three patients reported the early stages of an out-of-body experience. The study was discontinued but a similar one is being planned for a different group of patients.

Most recently, Drs. Bruce Greyson and Ian Stevenson at the University of Virginia received a large grant to support a cohort study of near-death experiencers and patients who were close to death at the same time but did not have a near-death experience. They will be studying the characteristics and factors involved in both sets of subjects to try to determine significant differences.

The Need for a New Paradigm

If, in fact, we have anomalous experiences that are not explainable by our current paradigms, we need to move forward to develop new rules, assumptions, and theories to support the investigation of these new phenomena. One of the first issues must be a description of the acceptable phenomena to be researched. The soul—or immaterial essence, as I would prefer to call it—should not be regarded as the purview of religious authorities and not appropriate for scientific inquiry. There is enough evidence that there is something else besides our physical being operating in humans that warrants scientific investigation.

The transition to studying the immaterial essence of man will not be easy. In 1957, Eileen Garrett, the famous medium and founder of the Parapsychological Library Foundation in New York, made the following comments concerning survival research that addresses the current attitude toward "soulful" research: "That we have the scientific mechanism for such exploration is true. The place of applied science is recognized, but what is needed for the new communication are explorers with imagination, persistence and curiosity. . . . There is an unspoken taboo . . . against discussing man's hope for life beyond death in objective terms. The scholar's disdain, the self-conscious intellectual's too-quick smile, and the minister's rolling phrases respect that taboo. They avoid rather than face the issue: they are designed to head off the unsophisticated questioner, the sincere investigator, the truly perplexed" (Anyoff, 1974).

Gallup would support Garrett's position that pursuing this type of research will not be easy. He found that scientists and physicians tended to be nonbelievers in life after death and other paranormal beliefs. When surveyed, only 16 percent of scientists said they believed in life after death, while 32 percent of physicians did. They, however, were far less convinced than the general adult public, 67 percent of whom believed in an afterlife. Only 8 percent of scientists believed in reincarnation. While only 9 percent of physicians held this belief, 23 percent of the general population believed in reincarnation. Only 5 percent of scientists and 9 percent of physicians believed it is possible to contact the dead, yet 24 percent of the general population think it is possible. Gallup also reported that the general population was more likely than the scientist and the physicians to have had actual experiences strengthening their beliefs (Gallup, 1982).

Our traditional research paradigms have been, as Harmon stated, based on several assumptions:

1. What is real is what we know, assisted and unassisted, through our five physical senses.

2. We can observe an object or event without causing it to change.

3. Knowing the smallest element is the key to understanding.

While these assumptions have been shown to be incorrect in many research endeavors, there are some questions related to the experiences described in this book that can be answered under that framework:

How does movement enhance consciousness?

What is the mechanism by which patients can hear but not move early in their unconscious experience?

What assessment tools can we use that detect awareness but no psycho-motor ability?

There are other questions, however, that need a different framework in order to answer them:

Why do patients have different types of experiences while unconscious?

What is the mechanism by which a person can have an inner dialogue yet not be aware of the external environment?

How do patients receive energy from others?

How does the positive energy help them get better?

How does negative energy deplete them?

What happens with the rare patient who is pronounced dead and then recovers?

What are the different forces or life systems that function within the body?

We need to make different assumptions about our research methods that enable us to answer these questions. William Harman suggests that in order to effectively study consciousness and para-normal experiences we need a holistic science which would have the following characteristics: "Present science, tremendously ef-fective in its chosen context, is based on an ontological assumption of separateness and an epistemological assumption of physical sense data as the sole empirical evidence on which the scientific picture of reality is to be based. The prospect of an extended science would build upon an ontological assumption of oneness, whole-ness, interconnectedness of everything and an epistemological choice to include all the evidence" (Harman, 1991, p. 17).

The following statements would guide us in this new paradigm:

1. What is real can be known directly or indirectly through manifestations in addition to our senses.

2. Any observation of an object under study can cause it to change.

3. The key to understanding can be achieved by knowing the unity of all the elements.
4. Subjective self-reports of trained experts are admissible.

Manifestations

Before we are able to objectify phenomena, we must first be able to observe manifestations of phenomena. Manifestations are like symptoms. They are not the root cause, but they indicate the presence of something else occurring. Curious, open-minded scientists look to those manifestations as indicators of doors to new discoveries. Manifestations are not measurable but often, as in the case of these extrasensory experiences, indicate the need for new types of measurements.

We also need to take into account the nature of the subjects and their state of being when observed and studied in a new field of investigation. For example, subjects, when they are out of their bodies, report a lack of concern for some of what was important to them in their usual state. The young mother who had an NDE during childbirth was ready to leave her husband and go with her mother who had died and was calling her. In her physical state, her husband was extremely important to her and would not have been dismissed so casually. Many subjects during the OBE studies reported not being interested in the research object when in the OBE state. Full of enthusiasm before the research, they often became disinterested in "checking out" the object when out of their bodies.

Lawrence LeShan talks about the unity principle to which mystics ascribe while in this state. He says that they all perceive the unity and harmony that exist in the altered state. It seems plausible that this view can be applied to designing a valid research approach. Subjects when out of their bodies seem to notice what is out of place—not in unity with their surroundings. We are not supposed to have shoes on roofs of hospitals or out on the ledges. In one of the studies the subject failed to see the research object but noticed a visitor who was in the research space when she was not supposed to be there. If we want to validate the perceptions of subjects while in altered states, we need to set up objects and/or situations that would be of interest to these subjects in those states, not what is of interest to them in their physical body state.

We also need a unitary view of man as a combination of the physical body and immaterial essence. Gary Zukav describes this new direction in the following manner: "We are evolving from five-sensory humans into multisensory humans. Our five senses together form a single sensory system that is designed to perceive physical reality. The perceptions of a multisensory human extend beyond physical reality to the larger dynamical systems of which our physical reality is a part. The multisensory human is able to perceive, and to appreciate, the role that our physical reality plays in a larger picture of evolution, and the dynamic by which our physical reality is created and sustained. This realm is invisible to the five-sensory human" (Zukav, 1989, p. 27).

This unitary view of man can only be achieved by consolidating the efforts of many disciplines. Historically, each discipline has designed research protocols that operate within the paradigms of the discipline. We have all been unsuccessful in truly explaining the true nature of human experiences. To be more effective, we need research teams that are made up of representatives of a variety of disciplines. We need an interdisciplinary approach to design meaningful research projects, one that is holistic in its orientation.

IMPLICATIONS FOR CLINICIANS

While more research is necessary in the field of consciousness to completely understand the nature of related experiences, there are some guidelines clinicians can use in caring for unconscious patients based on the information we currently have.

When someone is unconscious, it is important to treat that person as a person. All the subjects described how important it was to be treated as a person. They found much consolation in being talked to instead of about, being recognized as a person with particular likes and dislikes, being treated in a caring, emotionally supportive way. Recognizing the personhood of the patient helps him or her to maintain a sense of identity. It also helps lessen the confusion that patients experience in this unfamiliar environment.

Talk to the patients about what you are doing and what is generally happening to them. Patients reported being very disoriented and often misinterpreted what was being done by their caregivers. Because it is difficult to tell when the patient hears what is being said and what he remembers, it is important to constantly present the reality of the moment.

Encourage only emotionally positive friends and family members to see the patient. Most ICUs have visiting rules that limit visitors to the immediate family. This policy may not be the most advantageous for the patient since not all family members are caring and supportive. Sometimes the most emotionally significant person is a nonrelative. It is important for the caregivers and family members to remember that the purpose of hospitalization is to provide the treatment and environment that are optimal for the patient's survival and recovery. Having an abusive husband visit an unconscious patient is not going to help that patient. The visit may, in fact, be harmful. In one instance, I encouraged the ICU nurses to have a patient's golfing partner visit. He was one of the most emotionally significant persons to the patient.

Only those caregivers who have a positive emotional connection to the patients should provide care for them. The patients sense when a caregiver is detached or negative toward them. They also sense when someone genuinely cares about them. This genuine caring improves the quality of their existence and optimizes their chances for recovery.

After the patients recover, provide an opportunity for them to talk about their experiences. After waking up, the subjects often need to discuss what happened to them. A non-judgmental conversation about their experiences will improve the quality of their recovery. After the subjects described their experiences as part of this research project, they asked many questions about what happened to them. Some reported having nightmares for months. Many reported being told to keep quiet and not ask questions for fear of being thought of as crazy.

Normalize the experience for the patients. The most meaningful information I gave the patients was how many other patients had similar experiences. Even though I often did not know why a certain experience occurred, I could tell them about the other patients and their experiences. I also told them that having these experiences was not a sign of psychopathology. They often found that statement reassuring since it gave them the freedom to discuss what happened to them with others.

COMMENT

It is my hope that you, the reader, found the experiences of these patients fascinating. For me, listening to patients' descriptions of what happened while they were presumed to be unconscious was a humbling experience. With all our sophisticated technology and advanced understanding of the human body, there was little that prepared me for the variety and complexity of experiences reported by the patients.

APPENDIX

FURTHER EVIDENCE FOR VERIDICAL PERCEPTION DURING NEAR-DEATH EXPERIENCES*

Kenneth Ring and Madelaine Lawrence

Abstract: We briefly surveyed research designed to validate alleged out-of-body perceptions during near-death experiences. Most accounts of this kind that have surfaced since Michael Sabom's work are unsubstantiated self-reports or, as in claims of visual perception of blind persons, completely undocumented or fictional, but there have been some reports that were corroborated by witnesses. We briefly present and discuss three new cases of this kind.

What if you slept, and what if in your sleep you dreamed, and what if in your dream you went to heaven and there plucked a strange and beautiful flower, and what if when you awoke you had the flower in your hand?

Ah, what then?

Samuel Taylor Coleridge

Despite repeated expressions for the need to verify out-of-body perceptions during near-death experiences (NDEs) (for example, Blackmore, 1984, 1985; Cook, 1984; Holden, 1988, 1989; Holden and Joesten, 1990; Kincaid, 1985; and Krishnan, 1985), the last

*Published in the *Journal of Near-Death Studies*, 11(4), Summer, 1993, pp. 223–229.

decade has produced virtually nothing of substance on this vital issue. Michael Sabom's pioneering work (Sabom, 1981, 1982) is now recognized as virtually the only evidence from systematic research in the field of near-death studies that suggests NDErs can sometimes report visual perceptions that are physically impossible and not otherwise explicable by conventional means. To be sure, Sabom's data remain controversial, but the point is that they are still the only extensive body of evidence that bears on the question of veridical perception during near-death states.

Subsequent investigators, such as Janice Miner Holden and Leroy Joesten (1990), have attempted to follow Sabom's lead, but their work has been inconclusive, a casualty of various bureaucratic and methodological complications. What has emerged instead in the aftermath of Sabom's research is largely a miscellany of unsubstantiated self-reports as tantalizing as they are unverifiable. These reports dot the landscape of near-death studies like so many promising trails (Grey, 1985, pp. 37–38; Moody and Perry, 1988, pp. 134–135; and Ring, 1984, pp. 42–44), but efforts to pursue their tracks to definite conclusions almost always prove disappointing. This is particularly true for precisely those cases that hold out the greatest hope of confounding the challenge of skeptics, namely those where blind persons are alleged to have seen accurately during the NDEs.

For example, more than a decade ago, one of us (K. R.) learned of three such elusive cases from Fred Schoonmaker, one of the first physicians to conduct an extensive investigation of NDEs. In a telephone conversation Schoonmaker mentioned that he had come across three blind persons who had furnished him with evidence of veridical visual perceptions while out-of-body, including one woman he said had been congenitally blind. On hearing the details of this last story, I (K. R.) became very excited and urged him to publish an article on these extraordinary NDEs. Regrettably, he never did.

Another example of a blind person purportedly having detailed visual perception during an NDE was described by Raymond Moody and Paul Perry (1988, pp. 134–135). Intrigued to learn more about his case, not long ago I (K. R.) asked Moody to share with me some further particulars about its evidentiality. Unfortunately, he could only tell me that he had learned of this story as a result of another physician's playing a tape about it following one of Moody's lectures. He didn't remember the physician's name and therefore could do no more than relate the brief account his book attested to (R. A. Moody, Jr., personal communication, February, 1991).

Perhaps the most disappointing outcome of this kind of search was in response to the astonishing case of a woman named Sarah, with which still another physician, Larry Dossey, began a recent book (Dossey, 1989). According to Dossey, Sarah had had a cardiac arrest during gall bladder surgery, but had been successfully resuscitated. Upon recovery she had "amazed the. . . . surgery team" by reporting a clear, detailed memory of the operating room layout: the scribbles on the surgery schedule board in the hall outside, the color of the sheets covering the operating table, the hairstyle of the head scrub nurse . . . and even the trivial fact that her anesthesiologist that day was wearing unmatched socks. All this she knew even though she had been fully anesthetized and unconscious during the surgery and the cardiac arrest. But what made Sarah's vision even more momentous was the fact that, since birth, she had been blind (Dossey, 1989, p.18).

This sounds like the ideal case of its kind; and that, in a sense, is exactly what it is , in a different sense. Kindly responding to an inquiry for more information about this case, Dossey confessed to me (K. R.) that he had "constructed" it on the basis of a composite description of the out-of-body testimony of NDErs such as that found in Sabom's and Moody's books. With this example we seem to have come full circle, to where the mere lore of NDE veridicality subtly shades into a dangerous self-confirming proposition and to another dead end.

That skeptical conclusion is the impression left by this cursory review of the cases that have come to light since Sabom's trailblazing efforts. However, there have been some subsequent reports that seem to represent evidence that Dossey's fiction may in the end prove indeed to be substantiated NDE fact: the testimony of NDErs that has been supported by independent corroboration of witnesses.

Perhaps the most famous case of this kind is that of Maria, originally reported by her critical care social worker, Kimberly Clark (1984). Maria was a migrant worker who, while visiting friends in Seattle, had a severe heart attack. She was rushed to Harborview Hospital and placed in the coronary care unit. A few days later she had a cardiac arrest and an unusual out-of-body experience. At one point in this experience, she found herself outside the hospital and spotted a single tennis shoe sitting on the ledge of the north side of the third floor of the building. Maria not only was able to indicate the whereabouts of this oddly situated object, but was able to provide precise details concerning its appearance, such as that its little toe was worn and one of its laces was stuck underneath its heel. Upon hearing Maria's story, Clark, with some considerable degree of skepticism and metaphysical misgiving, went to the location described to determine whether any such shoe could be found. Indeed it was just where and precisely as Maria had described it, except that from the window through which Clark was able to see it, the details of its appearance that Maria had specified could not be discerned. Clark concluded that the only way she could have had such a perspective was if she had been floating right outside and at very close range to the tennis shoe. I retrieved the shoe and brought it back to Maria; it was very concrete evidence for me (Clark, p. 243).

Not everyone, of course, would concur with Clark's interpretation; but assuming the authenticity of the account, which we have no reason to doubt, the facts of the case seem incontestable. Maria's inexplicable detection of the inexplicable shoe is a strange and strangely beguiling sighting of the sort that has the power to arrest a skeptic's argument in mid-sentence, if only by virtue of its indisputable improbability. And yet it is only one case and, however discomfiting to some it might temporarily be, it can perhaps be conveniently filed away as merely a puzzling anomaly, in the hope that some prosaic explanation might someday be found.

Such a response is understandable and seems rational. However, there are more cases like Maria's, and we have found some. Since our search for conclusive cases of blind NDErs had thus far proven unavailing, we directed our efforts to tracking down instances of the "Maria's shoe" variety, where improbable objects in unlikely locations were described by NDErs and where at least one witness could either confirm or disprove the allegation. So far we have found the following three such cases, two of which, oddly enough, involve shoes!

CASE ONE

In 1985, Kathy Milne was working as a nurse at Hartford Hospital. Milne had already been interested in NDEs, and one day found herself talking to a woman who had been resuscitated and who had had an NDE. Following a telephone interview with me (K. R.) on August 24, 1992, she described the following account in a letter:

She told me how she floated up over her body, viewed the resuscitation effort for a short time and then felt herself being pulled up through several floors of the hospital. She then found herself above the roof and realized she was looking at the skyline of Hartford. She marvelled at how interesting this view was and out of the corner of her eye, she saw a red object. It turned out to be a shoe. She thought about the shoe. . . . and suddenly, she felt "sucked up" a blackened hole. The rest of her NDE was fairly typical, as I remember. I was relating this to a skeptical resident who in a mocking manner left. Apparently, he got a janitor to get him onto the roof. When I saw him later that day, he had a red shoe and became a believer too (K. Milne, personal communication, October 19, 1992).

One further comment about this second white crow, again in the form of a single, improbably situated shoe sighted in an external location of a hospital: After my (K. R.) initial interview with Milne, I made a point of inquiring whether she had ever heard of the case of Maria's shoe. Not only was she unfamiliar with it, but she was utterly amazed to hear of another story so similar to the one she had just recounted for me. It remains an unanswered question how these isolated shoes arrive at their unlikely perches for later viewing by astonished NDErs and their baffled investigators.

CASE TWO

In the summer of 1982, Joyce Harmon, a surgical intensive care unit (ICU) nurse at Hartford Hospital, returned to work after a vacation. On that vacation she had purchased a new pair of plaid shoelaces, which she happened to be wearing on her first day back at the hospital. That day, she was involved in resuscitating a patient, a woman she didn't know, giving her medicine. The resuscitation was successful, and the next day, Harmon chanced to see the patient, whereupon they had a conversation, the gist of which (not necessarily a verbatim account) is as follows (J. Harmon, personal communication, August 28, 1992):

> The patient, upon seeing Harmon, volunteered, "Oh, you're the one with the plaid shoelaces!"
> "What?" Harmon replied, astonished. She says she distinctly remembers feeling the hair on her neck rise.
> "I saw them," the woman continued. "I was watching what was happening yesterday when I died. I was up above."

CASE THREE

In the late 1980s, Sue Saunders was working at Hartford Hospital as a respiratory therapist. One day, she was helping to resuscitate a man in the emergency room, whose electrocardiogram had gone flat. Medics were shocking him repeatedly with no results. Saunders was trying to give him oxygen. In the middle of the resuscitation, someone else took over for her and she left.

A couple of days later, she encountered this patient in the ICU. He spontaneously commented, "You looked so much better in your yellow top."

She, like Harmon, was so shocked at this remark that she got goosebumps, for she had been wearing a yellow smock the previous day. "Yeah," the man continued, "I saw you. You had something over your face and you were pushing air into me. And I saw your yellow smock." Saunders confirmed that she had had something over her face—a mask—and that she had worn the yellow smock while trying to give him oxygen, while he was unconscious and without a heartbeat (S. Saunders, personal communication, August 28, 1992).

DISCUSSION

The three cases we have presented briefly attest to three important observations: (1) patients who claim to have out-of-body experiences while near death sometimes describe unusual objects that they could not have known about by normal means; (2) these objects can later be shown to have existed in the form and location indicated by the patient's testimony; and (3) hearing this testimony has a strong emotional and cognitive effect on the caregivers involved, either strengthening their pre-existing belief in the authenticity of NDEs or a kind of on-the-spot conversion.

We are not suggesting, of course, that the cases we have described here constitute proof of the authenticity of NDEs or even that they necessarily demonstrate that patients have been literally out of the bodies when they report what they do. We only submit that such cases add to the mounting evidence that veridical and conventionally inexplicable visual perceptions do occur during NDEs, and the fact of their existence needs to be reckoned with by near-death researchers and skeptics alike.

We hope that our small collection of cases will motivate other investigators to search for and document their own, so that this body of data will increase to the point where it becomes generally accepted, whatever its explanation may ultimately be. Until such time as more studies like those undertaken by Sabom and Holden are actually conducted by near-death researchers, or a genuine case of corroborated visual perception by a blind NDEr is reported, perhaps instances of the kind we have offered here will constitute the strongest argument that cases like Dossey's Sarah are by no means as fictional as skeptics might think.

REFERENCES

Blackmore, S. J. (1984). Are out-of-body experiences evidence for survival? Reply to Cook (Letter). *Journal of Near-Death Studies*, 4: 169–171.

Blackmore, S. J. (1985). Are out-of-body experiences evidence for survival? Reply to Krishnan (Letter). *Journal of Near-Death Studies*, 5(1): 79–82.

Clark, K. (1984). Clinical interventions with near-death experiencers. In B. Greyson and C. P. Flynn (eds.), *The Near-Death Experience: Problems, Prospects, Perspectives*, Springfield, IL: Charles C. Thomas, pp. 242–255.

Cook, E. W. (1984). Are out-of-body experiences evidence for survival? (Letter). *Journal of Near-Death Studies*, 4: 167–169.

Dossey, L. (1989). *Recovering the Soul: A Scientific and Spiritual Search*. New York: Bantam.

Grey, M. (1985). *Return from Death: An Exploration of the Near-Death Experience*. London: Arkana.

Holden, J. M. (1988). Visual perception during the naturalistic near-death out-of-body experience. *Journal of Near-Death Studies*, 7: 107–120.

Holden, J. M. (1989). Unexpected findings in a study of visual perception during the naturalistic near-death out-of-body experiences. *Journal of Near-Death Studies*, 7: 155–163.

Holden, J. M., and Joesten, L. (1990). Near-death veridicality research in the hospital setting: Problems and promise. *Journal of Near-Death Studies*, 9: 45–54.

Kincaid, W. M. (1985). Sabom's study should be repeated (Letter). *Journal of Near-Death Studies*, 5(2): 84–87.

Krishnan, V. (1985). Are out-of-body experiences evidence for survival? (Letter). *Journal of Near-Death Studies*, 5(1): 76–79.

Moody, R. A., Jr., and Perry, P. (1988). *The Light Beyond*. New York: Bantam.

Ring, K. (1984). *Heading Toward Omega: In Search of the Meaning of the Near-Death Experience*. New York: William Morrow.

Sabom, M. B. (1981). The near-death experience: Myth or reality? A methodological approach. *Journal of Near-Death Studies*, 1: 44–56.

Sabom, M. B. (1982). *Recollections of Death: A Medical Investigation*. New York: Harper and Row.

REFERENCES

Abram, H. S. (1965). Adaptation to open-heart surgery. *American J. Psychiat.*, 122: 659–667.

Alexander, F., and S. Selesnick (1966). *The History of Psychiatry.* New York: Harper and Row.

Alvarado, C. (1984). The physical detection of the astral body: An historical perspective. *Theta*, 8(2): 4–7.

Allen, D., and D. Nutt (1993). Co-existence of panic disorder and sleep paralysis. *Journal of Psychopharmacology*, 7(3): 293–294.

Anyoff, A. (1974). *Eileen Garrett and the World Beyond the Senses.* New York: William Morrow Publishers.

Arnette, J. K. (1992). On the mind/body problem: The theory of essence. *Journal of Near-Death Studies*, 11: 5–18.

Arnette, J. K. (1995). The theory of essence. II. An electromagnetic-quantum mechanical model of interactionism. *Journal of Near-Death Studies*, 13(2): 77–99.

Barrett, W. F. (1926). *Death Bed Visions.* London: Methuen.

Bartlett, L. (1978). Bernard Grad and energy. *Human Behavior*, June: 28–32.

Berger, H. (1929). Ueber das Elektrenkephalogramn desz Menschen. *Arch. Psychiatry*, 87: 527–570.

Blacher, R. (1971). Open-heart surgery: The patient's point of view. *Mount Sinai J. Med.*, 38: 74–78.

Blacher, R. (1972). The hidden psychosis of open-heart surgery. *JAMA*, 222(3): 305–308.

Blackmore, S. (1982). *Beyond the Body: An Investigation of Out-of-Body Experiences*. London: Heinemann.

Blackmore, S. (1993). *Dying to Live*. New York: Prometheus.

Bremer, F. (1936). Nouvelles recherches sur le mecanisme du sommeil. *Comp. Rend. Soc. Biol.*, 122: 460–464.

Brennan, B. A. (1987). *Hands of Lights: A Guide to Healing Through the Human Energy Field*. Toronto: Bantam Books.

Carr, D. B. (1981). Endorphins at the approach of death. *Lancet*, 1, 390.

Chorvinsky, M. (1992). Our strange world. *Fate*, 45(7): 31–35.

Chorvinsky, M. (1993). Our strange world. *Fate*, 46(5): 22–26.

Christopher, M. (1979). *Search for the Soul*. New York: Thomas Y. Crowell.

Clark, K. (1984). Clinical interventions with near-death experiencers. In B. Greyson and C. P. Flynn (eds.), *The Near-Death Experience: Problems, Prospects, Perspectives*. Springfield, IL: Charles C. Thomas.

Cobbe, F. (1882). *Peak in Darien Experiences*. London: Williams and Morgate.

Comer, N., L. Madow, and J. Dixon (1967). Observations of sensory deprivation in a life-threatening situation. *Amer. J. Psychiat*, 124(2): 164–169.

Crick, F. (1994). *The Astonishing Hypothesis: The Scientific Search for the Soul*. New York: Charles Scribner's Sons.

Crookall, R. (1961). *The Study and Practice of Astral Projection.*. London: Aquarian Press.

Crookall, R. (1964). *More Astral Projections*. London: Aquarian Press.

Crookall, R. (1972). *Casebook of Astral Projection*. Secaucus, NJ: University Books, 1972.

Damasio, A. (1994). *Descartes' Error*. New York: G. P. Putnam's Sons.

Darling, D. (1995). *Soul Search*. New York: Villard Books.

Dempsey, E. W., and R. S. Morison (1942). The production of rhythmically recurrent cortical potentials after localized thalamic stimulation. *Am. J. Physiology*, 135: 293–300.

Dennett, D. (1991). *Consciousness Explained*. Boston, MA: Little, Brown.

Descartes, R. (1986). *Meditations on First Philosophy* (J. Cottingham, Trans.). Cambridge, England: Cambridge University Press. (Original work published 1641.)

Dubin, W. R., H. L. Field, and B. S. Gasfriend (1979). Postcardiotomy delirium: A critical review. *J. Thorac. Card. Surg.*, 77: 586–594.

Easton, E., and F. MacKenzie (1988). Sensory-perceptual alterations: Delirium in the intensive care unit. *Heart and Lung,* 17: 229–237.

Eich, E., J. L. Reeves, and R. L. Katz (1985). Anesthesis, amnesia and the memory/awareness distinction. *Anesth. Analg.*, 64: 1143–1148.

Evans B. M. (1976). Patterns of arousal in comatose patients. *J. Neurol. Neurosurg. Psychiatr.*, 39: 392–402.

Frosch, J. (1983). *The Psychotic Process.* New York: International Universities Press, Inc.

Fukuda, K. (1993). One explanatory basis for the discrepancy of reported prevalences of sleep paralysis among health respondents. *Perceptual and Motor Skill*, 77(3): 803–807.

Gabbard, G., S. Twenlow, and F. Jones (1982). Do "near-death experiences" occur only near death? *Journal of Nervous and Mental Disease*, 169: 374–377.

Gallup, G. (1982). *Adventures in Immortality.* New York: McGraw-Hill.

Germine, M. (1991). Consciousness and synchronicity. *Medical Hypotheses*, 36: 277–283.

Gimenez, R. (1992). A metaphysical journey in a comatose state. *Clinical Nurse Specialist* 6(4): 191–194.

Godwin, M. (1994). *The Lucid Dreamer.* New York: Simon and Schuster.

Grad. B., R. J. Cadoret, and G. P. Paul (1961). The influence of an unorthodox method of treatment on wound healing in mice. *International Journal of Parapsychology*, 3: 5–24.

Greeley, A. (1975). *The Sociology of the Paranormal: A Reconnaissance.* Beverly Hills, CA: Sage Publications.

Green, C. (1968). *Out-of-Body Experiences.* London: Hamish Hamilton.

Greyson, B. (1981). Toward a psychological explanation of near-death experiences. *Journal of Near-Death Studies*, 1: 88–103.

Greyson, B. (1983a). The psychodynamics of near-death experiences. *Journal of Nervous and Mental Disease*, 171: 376–381.

Greyson, B. (1983b). The near-death experience scale: Construction reliability and validity. *Journal of Nervous and Mental Disease*, 171: 369–375.

Greyson, B. and N. Bush (1992). Distressing near-death experiences. *Psychiatry*, 55(1): 95–110.

Grof, S. (1976). *Realms of the Human Unconscious*. New York: E. P. Dutton.

Guyton, A. (1991). *Textbook of Medical Physiology*. Philadelphia: W. B. Saunders.

Harman, W. (1991). Does further progress in consciousness research await a reassessment of the metaphysical foundation of modern science? In K. Rao (ed.), *Cultivating Consciousness*. Westport, CT: Praeger.

Haynes, R. (1981). Faith healing and psychic healing: Are they the same? *Journal of Religion and Psychical Research*, 4(1): 22–29.

Heim, A. (1892). Remarks on fatal falls. *Swiss Alpine Club Yearbook*, 27: 327–337.

Helton, M. C., S. H. Gordon, and S. L. Nunnery (1980). The correlation between sleep deprivation and the intensive care unit psychosis. *Heart and Lung*, 13: 59–65.

Hobson, J. (1994). The Chemistry of Conscious States. Boston, MA: Little, Brown.

Howard, R. (1987). Incidents of auditory perception during anesthesia with traumatic sequelae. *Medical Journal of Australia*, 146: 44–46.

Hunt, M. (1993). *The Story of Psychology*. New York: Doubleday/Anchor Books.

Irwin, H. J. (1985). *Flight of Mind: A Psychological Study for the Out-of-Body Experience*. Metuchen, NJ.: Scarecrow Press.

Jennett, B., and G. Teasdale (1977). Aspects of coma after severe head injury. *Lancet*, 1: 878–881.

Kaplan H., and B. Sadock (1989). *Comprehensive Textbook of Psychiatry*. Baltimore: Williams and Wilkins.

Kastenbaum, R. (1978). *Between Life and Death*. New York: Springer.

Kornfeld, D. S, S. S. Heller, K. A. Frank, et al. (1978). Delirium after coronary artery bypass surgery. *J. Thoracic Cardiovascular Surg.*, 76: 93–96.

Krieger, D. (1979). *The Therapeutic Touch*. Englewood Cliffs, NJ: Prentice-Hall.

Kuhn, T. (1970). *The Structure of Scientific Revolutions*. Chicago, IL: University of Chicago Press.

Kurtz, P. (1988). Scientific evidence keeps us in the here and now. *Psychology Today*, 22(9): 15.

Lawrence, M. (1995a). The unconscious experience. *American Journal of Critical Care*, 4(3): 227–232.

Lawrence, M. (1995b). Paranormal experiences of previously unconscious patients. Proceedings of an International Conference: Parapsychology and Thanatology, 122–148.

LeShan, L. (1974). *The Medium, the Mystic, and the Physicist.* New York: Viking Press.

Lindal, E., et al. (1994). The qualitative difference of visions and visual hallucinations: A comparison of a general-population and clinical sample. *Compr.-Psychiatry,* 35(5): 405–408.

Loeb, L. (1981). *From Descartes to Hume.* Ithaca, NY: Cornell University Press.

Maslow, A. (1971). *The Farther Reaches of Human Nature.* New York: Viking Press.

Monroe, R. (1971). *Journeys Out of the Body.* New York: Doubleday.

Moody, R. A. (1975). *Life After Life.* Covington, GA: Mockingbird Books.

Moyers, Bill. (1993). *Healing and the Mind.* New York: Doubleday.

Muldoon, S. (1946). *The Case for Astral Projection.* Chicago: Aries Press.

Muldoon, S., and H. Carrington (1929). *The Projection of the Astral Body.* London: Rider.

Muldoon, S., and H. Carrington, (1951). *The Phenomena of Astral Projection.* London: Rider.

Myers, S. A., H. R. Austin, J. T. Grisson, and R. C. Nickeson (1983). Personality characteristics as related to the out-of-body experience. *Journal of Parapsychology*, 47: 131–144.

Neelon, V. (1990). Postoperative confusion. *Critical Care Nursing Clinics of North America*, 2(4): 579–587.

Noyes, R. (1972). The experience of dying. *Psychiatry*, 35: 174–184.

Noyes, R., and R. Kletti (1976). Depersonalization in the face of life-threatening danger. *Psychiatry*, 39: 19–27.

Nuland, S. (1995). *How We Die.* New York: Vintage Books.

Oiler, C. (1982). The phenomenological approach in nursing research. *Journal of Nursing Research*, 31: 178–181.

Olson, M. (1988). The incidence of out-of-body experiences in hospitalized patients. *Journal of Near-Death Studies*, 62(3): 169–174.

Ornstein, R. (1991). *The Evolution of Consciousness*. Englewood Cliffs, NJ: Prentice-Hall.

Osis, K. (1961). *Deathbed Observation by Physicians and Nurses*. New York: Parapsychology Foundation.

Osis, K. (1974). Out-of-body research at the American Society for Psychical Research. *ASPR Newsletter*, 1(27): 1–3.

Osis, K. and E. Haraldsson (1977). *At the Hour of Death*. New York: Avon.

Osis, K., and D. McCormick (1978). Insider's view of the OBE. *ASPR Newsletter*, July: 18–19.

Osis, K. and D, McCormick (1980). Kinetic effects at the ostensible location of an out-of-body projection during perceptual testing. *Journal of the American Society of Psychical Research*, 74: 319–329.

Palmer, J. (1978). The out-of body experience: A psychological theory. *Parapsychology Review*, 9(5): 19–22.

Palmer, J. (1979). A community mail survey of psychic experiences. *Journal of the American Society for Psychical Research*, 73: 221–251.

Panati, C. (1974). *Supersenses*. New York: Quadrangle Books.

Pelletier, K. (1985). *Toward a Science of Consciousness*. Berkeley, CA: Celestial Arts.

Penfield, W. (1955). The role of temporal cortex in certain psychical phenomena. *Journal of Mental Science*, 101: 451–465.

Persinger, M. A. (1993). Average diurnal changes in melatonin levels are associated with hourly incidence of bereavement apparitions: Support for the hypothesis of temporal (limbic) lobe microseizuring. *Perceptual and Motor Skills*, 76: 444–446.

Persinger, M. A., and S. Fisher (1990). Elevated, specific temporal lobe signs in a population engaged in psychic studies. *Perceptual and Motor Skills*, 71: 817–818.

Persinger, M. A., and K. Makarec (1992). The feeling of a presence and verbal meaningfulness in context of temporal lobe function: Factor analytic verification of the muses? *Brain and Cognition*, 20: 217–226.

Plum, F., and J. B. Posner (1982). *The Diagnosis of Stupor and Coma*. Philadelphia: F. A. Davis.

Podurgiel, M. (1990). The unconscious experience: A pilot study. *J. Neurosci. Nurs.*, 22: 52–53.

References   181

Ring, K. (1980). *Life at Death: A Scientific Investigation of the Near-Death Experience.* New York: Coward, McCann and Geoghegan.

Ring, K., and M. Lawrence (1993). Further evidence for veridical perception during near-death experiences. *Journal of Near-Death Studies,* Summer, 223–229.

Ring, K., and C. Rosing (1990). The omega project: an empirical study of the NDE-prone personality. *Journal of Near-Death Studies,* 8(4): 211–239.

Rodin, E. (1989). Comments on "A neurobiological model for near-death experiences." *Journal of Near-Death Studies,* 7(4): 255–259.

Rogers, C. (1961). *On Becoming a Person.* Boston: Houghton Mifflin.

Rogers, M. (1986). Science of unitary human beings. In V. M. Malinsky, *Explorations on Martha Rogers' Science of Unitary Human Beings.* Norwalk, CT: Appleton-Century-Crofts.

Rogo, S. (1984). Researching the out-of-body experience: the state of the art. *Journal of Near-Death Studies,* 4: 21–49.

Roll, W. (1995). General Discussion Day One. Proceedings of an International Conference: Parapsychology and Thanatology. New York: Parapsychology Foundation.

Saavedrea-Aguilar, J., and J. Gomez-Jeria (1989). A neurobiological model for near-death experience. *Journal of Near-Death Studies,* 7(4): 205–222.

Sabom, M. (1982). *Recollections of Death.* New York: Harper and Row.

Sadwin, A., et al. (1993). Post-traumatic headache syndrome. In S. Mandel et al. (eds.), *Minor Head Trauma.* New York: Springer-Verlag.

Sanders, P. (1989). *You Are Psychic.* New York: Fawcett Columbia.

Schnaper, N. (1975). The psychological implications of severe trauma: Emotional sequelae to unconsciousness. *Journal of Trauma,* 15: 94–98.

Serdahly, W. (1990). Thomas Kuhn revisited: Near-death studies and paradigm shifts. *Journal of Near-Death Studies,* 9(1): 5–10.

Sidgwick, H., and Committee (1984). Report on the census of hallucinations. Proceedings of the Society for Psychical Research, 10: 25–422.

Sperry, R. W. (1961). Cerebral organization and behavior. *Science,* 133: 1749–1757.

Sperry, R. W. (1962). Some general aspects of interhemisphere integration. In V. B. Mountcarth (ed.), *Interhemispheric Relations and Cerebral Dominance*. Baltimore: Johns Hopkins Press, Chap. 3, 43–49.

Tart, C. (1968). Psycho-physiological study of out-of-body experience in a selected subject. *Journal of the American Society for Psychical Research*, 62: 3–27.

Tosch P. (1988). Patients' recollections of their posttraumatic coma. *J. Neuroscience Nursing*, 20: 223–228.

Troost, B., and L. Hutchings (1989). Eye movements in loss of consciousness. *Bull. Soc. Beige Ophthalmol.*, 237: 209–226.

Tyrrell, G.N.M. (1953). *Apparitions*. London: Duckworth.

van Kaam, A. L. (1966). *Existential Foundations of Psychology*. Pittsburgh: Dusquesne University Press.

Wilson, I. (1987). *The After Death Experience*. New York: Quill.

Zukav, G. (1989). *The Seat of the Soul*. New York: Simon & Schuster.

INDEX

About the Author

MADELAINE LAWRENCE is Assistant Professor at the College of Education, Nursing and Health Professions, University of Hartford, West Hartford, Connecticut.

ISBN 0-275-95323-8

90000>

EAN

9 780275 953232

HARDCOVER BAR CODE